Diabetic diet after 50

75 Mouthwatering Low-Carb Recipes for Seniors Over 50 Striving towards a Healthier Diabetic Diet with 28-Day Meal Plan

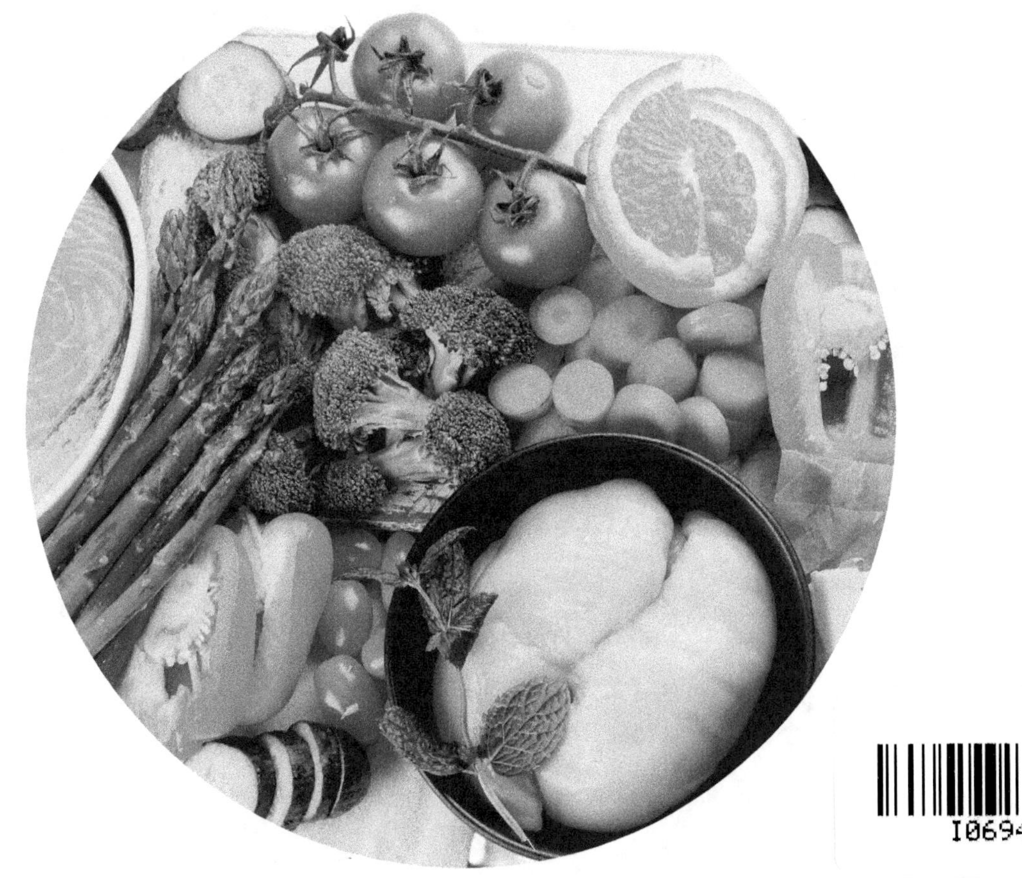

By Michelle Rockwell

Disclaimer

I, Michelle Rockwell, RDN, am a Registered Dietitian Nutritionist with a passion for transforming lives through the power of nutrition. The information provided in this book reflects my professional expertise and dedication to empowering individuals with the knowledge needed to make informed decisions about their health.

While every effort has been made to ensure the accuracy and completeness of the information presented, I cannot guarantee that the content is free from errors or omissions. Readers are advised to consult with their healthcare professionals before making any significant changes to their diet or lifestyle based on the information provided in this book.

The dietary plans and advice offered are designed to be general in nature and may not be suitable for everyone. Individual health conditions, preferences, and circumstances vary, and it is recommended that readers seek personalized guidance from qualified healthcare professionals for their specific needs.

I disclaim any liability, loss, or risk incurred as a consequence, directly or indirectly, of the use and application of any content of this book. The information in this book is not intended to replace professional medical advice, diagnosis, or treatment. I do not endorse any specific products or brands mentioned in this book.

Any mention of products or services is for informational purposes only and does not constitute an endorsement.

This book is meant to provide general guidance and inspiration on the topics of nutrition and health, and it is the readers' responsibility to use their judgment and seek professional advice as needed.

About the Author

I'm Michelle Rockwell, a dedicated Registered Dietitian Nutritionist (RDN) with a passion for transforming lives through the power of nutrition. With years of experience in this field, I take immense pride in helping individuals overcome their nutritional challenges and achieve a healthier, more balanced lifestyle. My journey into the world of nutrition began with a Bachelor's degree in Nutrition and Dietetics, where I delved deep into the science behind food and its impact on our well-being. I have since pursued advanced certifications in specialized areas, making me a well-rounded expert capable of tackling a wide range of nutritional concerns. As a clinical problem-solver, my approach is rooted in personalized care. I take the time to understand each client's unique circumstances, including their preferences, medical conditions, and lifestyle, to design tailored dietary plans that suit their needs. My goal is not just to provide quick fixes but to empower individuals with the knowledge they need to make informed choices for lasting results.

Table of contents

Table of contents

INTRODUCTION

Heather, a woman in her early 50s, had recently been diagnosed with Type 2 diabetes. Her initial response was a mix of confusion, fear, and uncertainty. The whirlwind of emotions that follows such a diagnosis is something many of us can empathize with. That's where I, as her counselor, stepped in.

Heather's first visit was filled with questions and doubts. She was overwhelmed by the prospect of completely changing her lifestyle and eating habits. I listened to her fears, and instead of bombarding her with facts and figures, I shared stories of others who had walked a similar path. These stories helped Heather understand that she wasn't alone and that change was possible. I knew that knowledge is power, especially when it comes to diabetes. I explained to Heather the fundamentals of diabetes, the role of carbohydrates, the importance of portion control, and the significance of incorporating fiber-rich foods into her diet. Together, we discussed the glycemic index and its impact on blood sugar.

I also emphasized that this wasn't about deprivation; it was about making informed, healthier choices. We explored delicious recipes and meal ideas that fit within her dietary needs. Heather's journey wasn't without its challenges. There were times when she felt discouraged, but we worked through them together. Slowly but steadily, she embraced the changes, choosing nutrient-packed foods and creating a balanced plate at each meal.

With each passing week, Heather began to see positive changes. Her blood sugar levels stabilized, and she had more energy. She no longer feared her diagnosis; instead, she took control of her health. Fast forward a few months, and Heather was a new woman. She had shed some excess weight, her blood pressure had improved, and her smile was infectious. The newfound energy allowed her to enjoy life more fully.

Heather's journey is a testament to the power of knowledge, support, and determination. With the right guidance and the willingness to embrace change, anyone can navigate the challenges of diabetes. Her transformation serves as a source of inspiration for others facing similar health concerns, proving that a diabetic diet isn't a sentence but a path to a healthier, happier life.

If Heather's story has resonated with you, know that you have the power to make similar changes in your own life or help someone else on their journey. It all begins with a single step, a desire for change, and the right support system.

About This Cookbook

Welcome to a gastronomic adventure that not only tempts your taste senses but also promotes your health. This cookbook is more than simply a compilation of recipes; it's a lifeline for anyone over the age of 50 dealing with the problems of diabetes.

You'll find a treasure trove of delectable, diabetes-friendly foods meticulously prepared to keep your blood sugar in balance and your taste buds thrilled within these pages. This cookbook, however, is more than a cookbook; it is a source of empowerment, a light of hope, and a testament to the transformational power of food. We've poured our hearts and souls into developing a cookbook that is both educational and incredibly personal. This cookbook will be your valued companion whether you are going on this path yourself or assisting a loved one.

You'll discover everything you need to make excellent, balanced meals in the following chapters, including:

- Diabetes and nutrition expert insights.
- Meal planning advice suited to your specific needs
- A diabetic meal plan designed to make your life simpler for 30 days.
- A wide range of dishes for breakfast, dessert, salad, soup, and even main dishes are available.
- Tips for living a healthy, satisfying life beyond 50.

We believe in the power of educated decision-making, and this cookbook is your passport to a better, happier life. So, turn the pages, relish the recipes, and soak in the knowledge. It's time to start on a health and gastronomic adventure. Your transformational journey begins here.

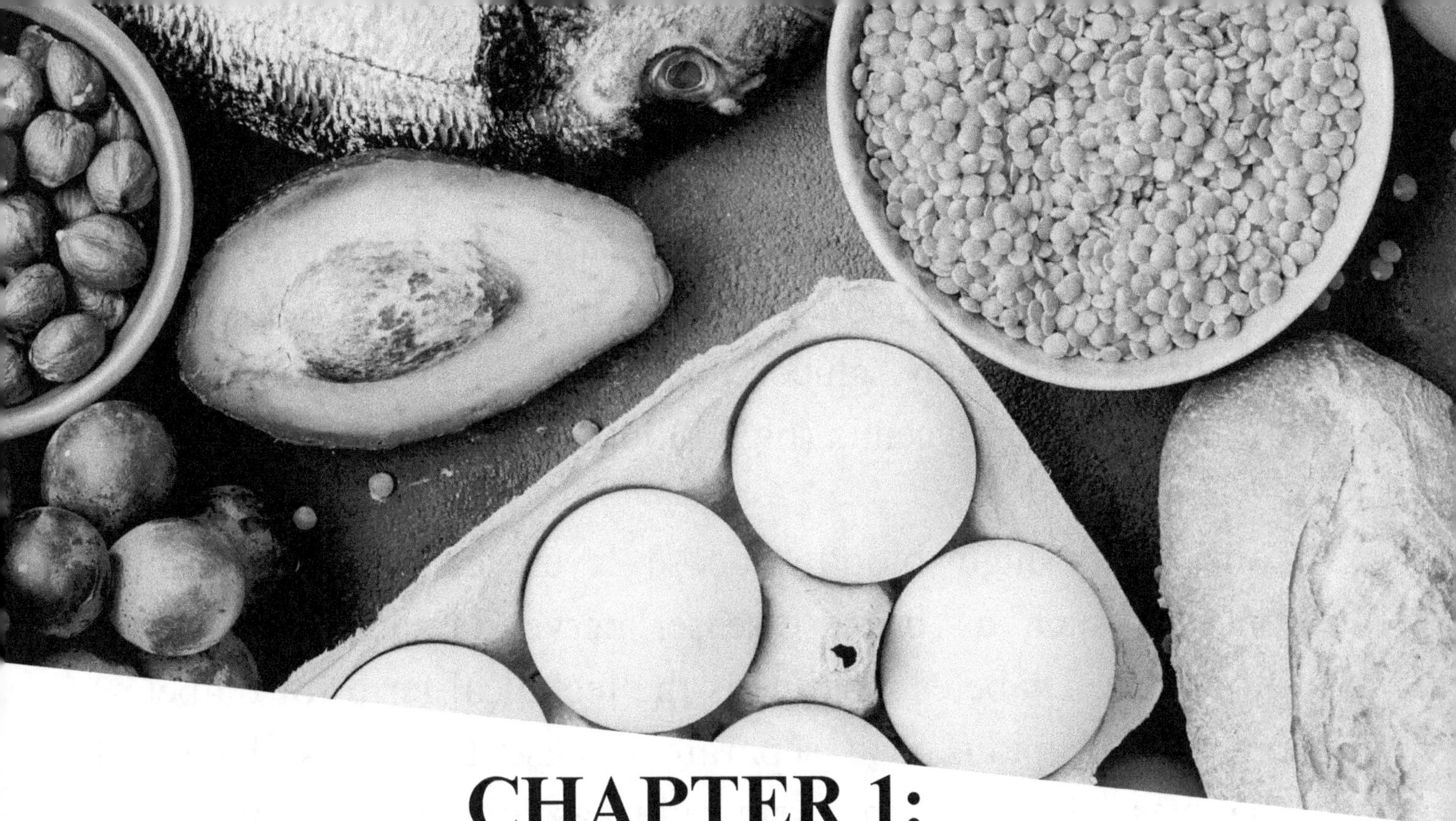

CHAPTER 1:
THE BASICS OF DIABETES AND NUTRITION

<u>What is Diabetes?</u>

Diabetes is a medical condition in which your blood sugar (glucose) levels are abnormally high. It occurs when your pancreas does not produce enough insulin, or none at all, or when your body does not adequately respond to the effects of insulin. People of all ages are affected by diabetes. Diabetes is a chronic (lifelong) disease that can be controlled with drugs and/or lifestyle adjustments.

Glucose (sugar) is mostly derived from carbs in food and beverages. It is your body's primary energy source. Your blood transports glucose to all of your body's cells, where it is used as energy.

When glucose enters your bloodstream, it needs assistance – a "key" – to achieve its destination. Insulin is a hormone. If your pancreas does not produce enough insulin or your body does not use it effectively, glucose builds up in your bloodstream, producing hyperglycemia (high blood sugar).

Consistently high blood glucose levels can lead to health concerns such as heart disease, nerve damage, and vision difficulties. Diabetes mellitus is the technical term for diabetes. Diabetes insipidus is a separate disease that uses the word "diabetes." They are both referred to as "diabetes" because they produce excessive thirst and frequent urination.

<u>Types of Diabetes</u>

Most common types of diabetes are;

1. Type 2 diabetes: This condition is characterized by insufficient insulin production and/or abnormal insulin cellular response (insulin resistance). The most prevalent kind of diabetes is this one. Although it primarily affects adults, children can also be affected. The period before Type 2 diabetes is known as prediabetes. Though they are higher than usual, your blood glucose levels are not high enough to receive a Type 2 diabetes diagnosis.
2. Type 1 diabetes is an autoimmune condition in which, for unclear reasons, your immune system targets and kills the insulin-producing cells in your pancreas.

Approximately 10% of individuals with diabetes have Type 1. Though it can manifest at any age, children and young people are often the ones diagnosed with it.

3. Gestational diabetes: This kind of diabetes during pregnancy. After pregnancy, gestational diabetes often disappears. On the other hand, if you have gestational diabetes, your chances of subsequently getting Type 2 diabetes are increased.

<u>Different types of Diabetes</u>

1. Diabetes that develops during the first six months of life is known as neonatal diabetes. It is a kind of monogenic diabetes as well. Permanent neonatal diabetes mellitus, a lifelong form of the disease, affects around 50% of newborns with diabetes. For the other half, the illness goes away within a few months after beginning, however it may recur at a later age. We refer to this as transitory diabetes mellitus in neonates.
2. Latent autoimmune diabetes (LADA): Similar to Type 1 diabetes, LADA is caused by an autoimmune response, but it progresses far more slowly. Typically, those with a LADA diagnosis are older than thirty.
3. Type 3c diabetes: This kind of diabetes is caused by injury to the pancreas that reduces its capacity to make insulin and is not related to an autoimmune disease. Diabetes is caused by pancreatic damage, which can be brought on by

hemochromatosis, pancreatic malignancy, pancreatitis, and cystic fibrosis. Type 3c is also brought on by pancreatectomy, or the removal of the pancreas.

<u>Blood Sugar Monitoring</u>

Regular blood sugar monitoring is essential for diabetes treatment. A glucometer is a gadget used to measure blood sugar. A little needle called a lancet can be used to puncture a fingertip. Then, in the glucometer, you deposit a drop of blood on a test strip to obtain a blood sugar level.

Blood sugar levels should be tested before meals and before going to bed. Continuous glucose monitoring (CGM) is an alternative that removes the need for finger sticks and may assess blood sugars in real time as frequently as every five minutes.

The American Diabetes Association (ADA) recommends the following blood sugar values as a general guideline:

Before meals, take 80 to 130 milligrams per deciliter (mg/dL) or 4.4 to 7.2 millimoles per liter (mmol/L).

Two hours after meals, less than 180 mg/dL (10.0 mmol/L).

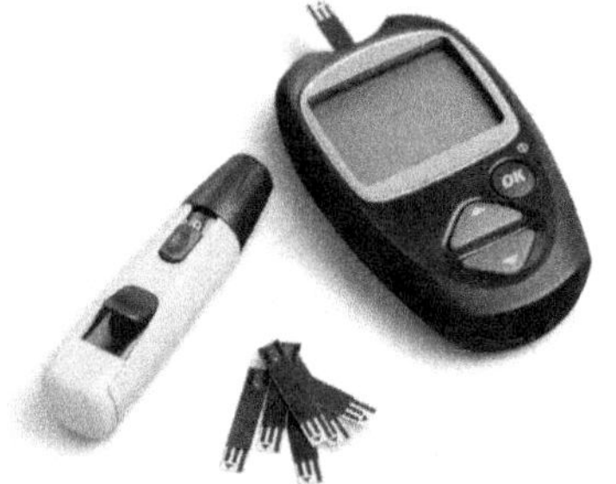 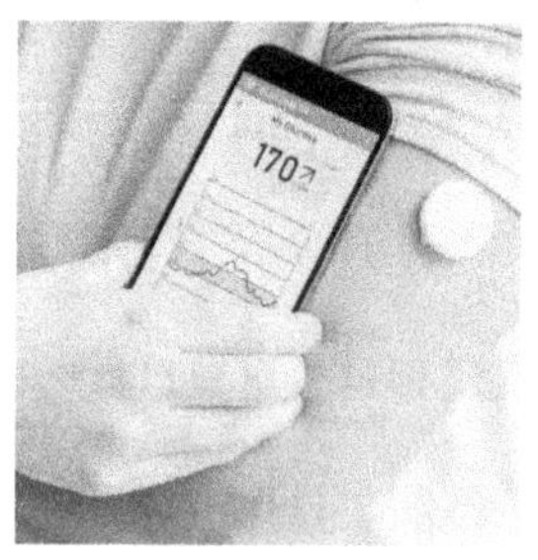 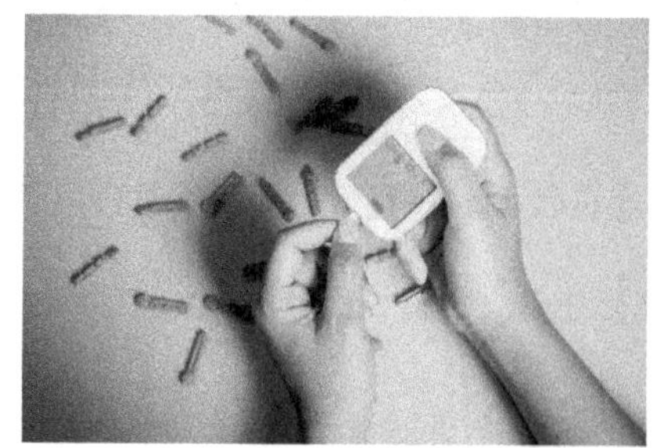

Importance of Nutrition

Nutrition is the foundation of good health and happiness. It is essential during all phases of life, from childhood to old age. Nutrition is very important for older people, and it is even more important for those who are managing chronic diseases like diabetes. Here are some of the reasons why nutrition is important, especially in the context of diabetes in older adults:

1. Blood Sugar Control: Maintaining stable blood sugar levels is critical for diabetics. The quality and quantity of carbs ingested, in particular, has a direct influence on blood sugar regulation. Making intelligent dietary choices can aid in the prevention of blood sugar spikes and crashes.

2. Energy and Vitality: Proper diet provides the energy required for everyday tasks, as well as the maintenance of muscle mass and general vitality. Age-related changes in metabolism and muscle mass may occur in older persons, making a balanced diet even more important for preserving strength and energy.

3. Diabetes complications might be exacerbated by being overweight. A healthy diet can aid in weight management, lowering the risk of obesity-related comorbidities and improving diabetes control overall.

4. Heart Disease: Heart disease is a big worry for diabetics. A heart-healthy diet high in fruits, vegetables, whole grains, and lean meats can help control cholesterol and lower the risk of cardiovascular problems.

5. Gut Health: A fiber-rich diet rich in whole grains, fruits, and vegetables promotes gut health. Better blood sugar management and general well-being are linked to good gut health.

6. Mineral and vitamin intake: Nutrient-rich meals provide essential vitamins and minerals that help with a variety of body processes. Specific minerals, such as calcium and vitamin D, may be required for bone health in older persons, and a well-balanced diet ensures that these requirements are satisfied.

7. Immune Function: A healthy immune system is supported by a proper diet. Maintaining a healthy immune response is critical for older persons to avoid infections and diseases.

8. Cognitive Function: According to research, a balanced diet may help people maintain cognitive function as they age. It is claimed that a diet high in antioxidants and healthy fats benefits brain function.

9. Digestive Health: Digestive difficulties are common in older persons, and a diet rich in fiber and probiotics can help keep the digestive tract healthy.

10. Quality of Life: Eating healthily is about more than simply avoiding health problems; it's also about having a better quality of life. A diversified and balanced diet gives a variety of flavors and textures that can enhance the enjoyment and satisfaction of meals.

11. Nutrition can have an impact on one's mood and emotional well-being. A well-balanced diet can help reduce blood sugar variations, which can cause mood swings and irritation.

Fiber and Diabetes

What exactly is fiber?

Dietary fiber is a carbohydrate found in plants. It is not absorbed or digested by the body, although it is vital to optimal health. Dietary fiber is classified into two types: soluble and insoluble. Most meals include both sorts, although one form is generally more abundant than the other.

Soluble Fiber;

Oats, oat bran, linseeds, barley, fruits and vegetables, nuts, beans, soya, and lentils are all high in this nutrient.

Insoluble Fiber;

Whole-meal bread, bran, whole-grain cereals, nuts, seeds, and the peel of several fruits and vegetables are good sources.

What is the significance of fiber?

Diabetes raises your chances of developing cardiovascular disease. Increased fiber consumption, particularly cereal and wholegrains, has been shown to lower the risk of cardiometabolic disorders (including cardiovascular disease, insulin resistance, and obesity) and colo-rectal cancer. Consuming more oat bran lowers cholesterol and blood pressure.

Dietary fiber absorbs liquids and increases the bulk of waste matter, resulting in softer, easier-to-pass stools. Soluble fiber-rich foods play a special function in lowering blood cholesterol. Increasing your dietary fiber intake can also aid with weight management.

These meals are full, and the majority have a lower glycemic index (GI), which can help you regulate your hunger and have a reduced impact on your blood glucose levels.

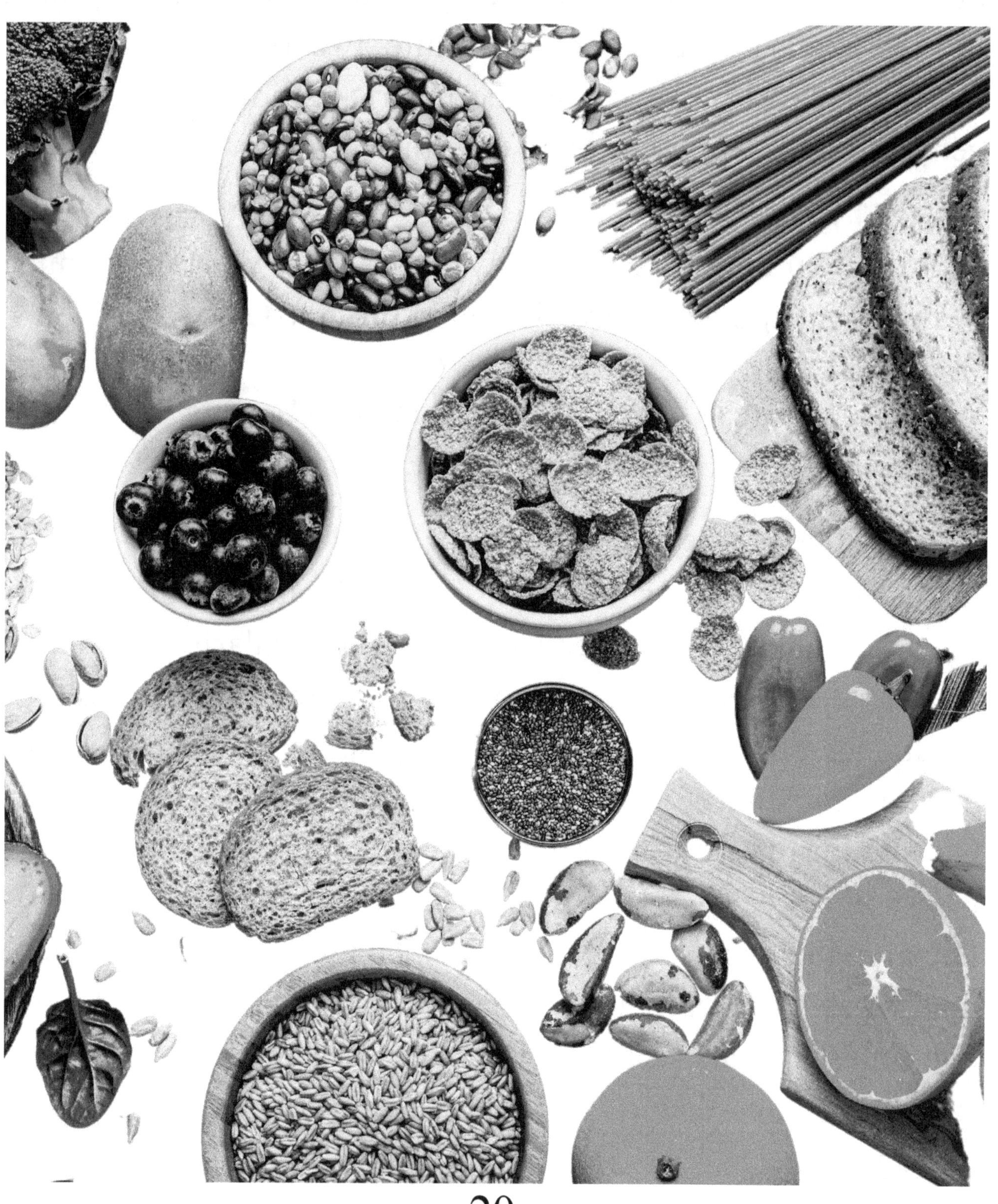

CHAPTER 2: MEAL PLANNING FOR DIABETES AFTER 50

Creating a Balanced Plate

The majority of the plate should be made up of non-starchy veggies. Spinach, carrots, lettuce, green beans, tomatoes, mushrooms, peppers, and so on are some examples. These foods are low in carbs but high in vitamins, minerals, and fiber, making them an important and nutritious element of diabetic diet.

Carbohydrate meals should be included in at least one of the quarter portions. Whole grain foods (breads, cereal, rice, and pasta), starchy vegetables (corn, potatoes, peas, and winter squash), dry beans and legumes (kidney, black, pinto), dairy foods (milk, yogurt, and milk substitutes such as soy milk), and fruit (fresh, juiced, or dried) are further examples. These meals are high-nutrients that feed our brain, kidneys, heart, and nervous system; some also include fiber, which promotes digestion. However, carbohydrate items should be minimized since they have the greatest impact on blood glucose levels.

Lean animal and plant-based proteins should make up the other minor part. Fish, seafood (shrimp, clams, oyster, crab, or mussels), lean cuts of beef or pig, eggs, low-fat cheese, and cottage cheese are all good sources of animal protein.

To help finish your meal, add a low-calorie drink such as water, unsweetened tea, or coffee.

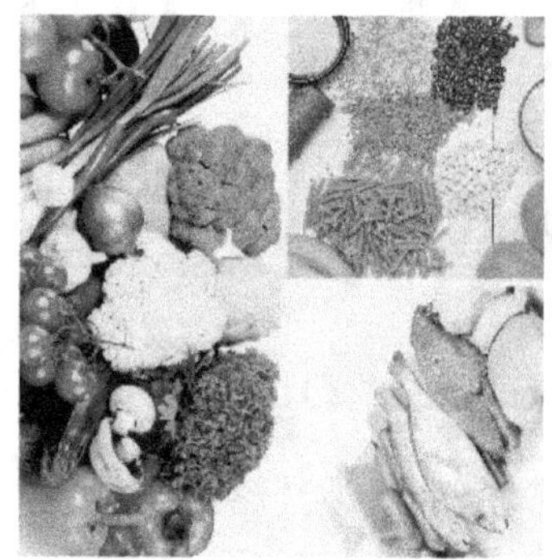

<u>Glycemic Index and Food Choices</u>

The GI is a grading system that assesses carbohydrates on a range of 1 to 100 depending on how much they elevate blood sugar. Breads, cake, and cookies have a high GI, but complete foods like unrefined grains, non-starchy vegetables, and fruits have a lower GI.

The GI values are classified into three categories. A food with a low GI will not elevate your blood sugar as much as a food with a medium or high GI;

- Low GI: 55 or less
- Medium GI: 56 to 69
- High GI: 70 to 100

Low-GI Foods (55 or Less)
Apple, Banana, Barley, Carrots(boiled), Chickpeas, Chocolate, Dates, Ice cream, Kidney beans, Lentils, Mango, Orange, Plantain, Rice noodles, Rolled oats, Skim milk, Soy milk, Spaghetti(white), Sweet corn, Vegetable soup.

Medium-GI Foods (56 to 69)

Brown rice(boiled), Couscous, French fries, Pineapple, Popcorn, Potato chips, Pumpkin(boiled),Sweet potato(boiled), Wheat flake biscuits cereal.

High-GI Foods (70 to 100)

Cornflakes, Instant oatmeal, Potato(boiled), Unleavened wheat bread, Watermelon, White rice(boiled), White bread (wheat), Whole wheat bread.

Understanding GI might help you figure out which foods are ideal for glucose management because carbs in meals boost blood sugar.

Reading Food Labels

It's not simple to decipher nutritional information on labels and packaging. I can help, which is wonderful news. These food labels are very handy if you plan your meals using carb counting!

1. Serving size

Examine the serving size first. The serving size specified is the basis for all of the information on the label. You will consume more calories, carbs, and other nutrients if you eat more than what is specified.

2. Amount per serving

The total amount of each nutrient in a single serving of the product is listed on the label's left side. Compare the labels of comparable foods using these numbers.

3. Calories

Consider calories as the amount of energy your body utilizes and consumes for daily activities.

4. Total carbohydrate

The term "total carbohydrate" on the label refers to the combined amount of sugar, starch, and fiber. Utilizing the total grams is crucial when calculating carbohydrates or selecting which food to include.

5. Added sugar

Sugar is one of three forms of carbohydrates found in food. Added sugar helps to distinguish between sugar that exists naturally in food (such as yogurt or fruit) and sugar that was added during processing (such as cookies, candies, and soda).

6. Fiber

The component of plant meals known as fiber is either not digested or, in other cases, is only partially digested. Good sources of dietary fiber include whole intact grains, fruits, vegetables, and dried beans like kidney or pinto beans.

7. Sugar alcohols

Sugar alcohols are sugar substitutes with less calories per gram than sugars and starches. Sugar alcohols include sorbitol, xylitol, and mannitol. If a food includes sugar alcohols, it will be indicated under Total Carbohydrate on the label. It's crucial to remember that meals containing sugar alcohols aren't always low in carbs or calories. Furthermore, just because a container says "sugar-free" on the front does not imply that it is calorie or carbohydrate-free. Always check the label for total carbohydrate grams and calories.

8. Fats

Total fat indicates how much fat is in one dish of food. To minimize your risk of heart disease, attempt to substitute foods high in saturated fat or trans fat with those rich in monounsaturated and polyunsaturated fats.

9. Sodium

The scientific name for salt is sodium. It has no effect on blood sugar. Excess dietary salt, on the other hand, raises your risk of high blood pressure and heart disease. You can taste the saltiness of some meals, such as pickles or bacon. However, concealed salt may be found in a variety of meals, including salad dressings, lunch meat, canned soups, and other packaged foods. Reading labels can assist you in locating these hidden sources and comparing the salt content of various items. Whether you have diabetes or not, the standard recommended is 2300 milligrams (mg) or fewer per day.

10. List of ingredients

Ingredient lists may be quite useful. The ingredients are given in weight order, with the first item containing the most of the meal. Knowing the components can help you make healthier choices, such as boosting fiber or lowering sugar.

Nutrition Facts
Valeur nutritive

Per 1 cup (250 mL) / par 1 tasse (250 mL)

Amount Teneur	% Daily Value % valeur quotidienne
Calories / Calories 80	
Fat / Lipides 0 g	**0 %**
Saturated / saturés 0 g + Trans / trans 0 g	**0 %**
Cholesterol / Cholestérol 0 mg	
Sodium / Sodium 115 mg	**5 %**
Carbohydrate / Glucides 12 g	**4 %**
Fibre / Fibres 0 g	**0 %**
Sugars / Sucres 11 g	
Protein / Protéines 9 g	
Vitamin A / Vitamine A	15 %
Vitamin C / Vitamine C	0 %
Calcium / Calcium	30 %
Iron / Fer	0 %
Vitamin D / Vitamine D	45 %

CHAPTER 3: A 28-DAY MEAL PLAN
Week 1

	Breakfast	Lunch	Dessert	Dinner
Day 1	Breakfast Salad with Egg & Salsa Verde Vinaigrette	Greek Salmon Salad with Tahini Yogurt Dressing	Low-Carb Chocolate Greek Yogurt Ice Cream	Chicken Casserole
Day 2	Spinach & Egg Scramble with Raspberries	Cucumber and Tomato Salad	Lemon Blueberry Cupcakes	Oven Roasted Turkey breast
Day 3	Skillet Veggie and Egg Scramble	Spinach and Chickpea Salad	Coconut Milk Shake	Baked Chicken with Onions & Leeks
Day 4	Low Carb Cottage Cheese Pancakes	Broccoli and cranberry salad	Greek Yogurt Berry Popsicles	Turkey meatballs with zucchini noodles
Day 5	Protein Pancakes	Spinach and Berry Salad	Spiced Pumpkin Cookies	Grounded Beef with Vegetable Stir-fry
Day 6	Oatmeal with Fruit & Nuts	Roasted beet and orange salad	Low-carb berry chia pudding	Lemon Pepper Chicken
Day 7	Banana Pancakes	Roasted Vegetable Salad	Strawberry-Mango Nice Cream	Garlic Chicken thighs

Week 2

	Breakfast	Lunch	Dessert	Dinner
Day 8	Blackberry Cinnamon Muffins	Chicken and Rice Soup	Greek Yogurt Berry Popsicles	Fish Tacos with Avocado Salsa
Day 9	Low Carb Cottage Cheese Pancakes	Turkey & Barley Soup	Sugar-free Coconut Macaroons	Garlic Tiger Shrimp
Day 10	Apple Walnut Pancakes	Cabbage and Sausage Soup	Coconut Milk Shake	Grilled Tuna Steaks with Cilantro and Basil
Day 11	Chocolate Chia Seed Pudding with Almond Milk	Quinoa and Vegetable Soup	Low-carb berry chia pudding	Baked salmon with mayonnaise
Day 12	Bagel Avocado Toast	Spicy Chicken Noodle Soup with Soft-Boiled Eggs	Greek Yogurt Berry Popsicles	Grilled Salmon with Avocado Salsa
Day 13	Banana Pancakes	Mexican Beef Stew	Cinnamon baked apples	One-Pot Garlic Shrimp & Broccoli
Day 14	Breakfast Salad with Egg & Salsa Verde Vinaigrette	Slow-Cooker Vegetable Minestrone Soup	Lemon Blueberry Cupcakes	Lemon Pepper Baked Catfish

Week 3

	Breakfast	Lunch	Dessert	Dinner
Day 15	Breakfast Salad with Egg & Salsa Verde Vinaigrette	Mediterranean Chickpea Salad	Greek Yogurt Berry Popsicles	Balsamic Chicken
Day 16	Chocolate Chia Seed Pudding with Almond Milk	Shrimp Scampi	Sugar-free Coconut Macaroons	Grounded Beef with Vegetable Stir-fry
Day 17	Bagel Avocado Toast	Brown Rice and Vegetable Stir-fry	Spiced Pumpkin Cookies	Garlic Chicken thighs
Day 18	Blackberry Cinnamon Muffins	Tortilla Chip Flounder with Black Bean Salad	Low-carb berry chia pudding	Oven Roasted Turkey breast
Day 19	Protein Pancakes	Pasta Puttanesca with Beef	Banana Oatmeal Cookies	Lemon Pepper Chicken
Day 20	Oatmeal with Fruit & Nuts	Spaghetti with Tomato and Basil	Cinnamon baked apples	Turkey meatballs with zucchini noodles
Day 21	Skillet Veggie and Egg Scramble	Cauliflower Rice	Strawberry-Mango Nice Cream	Chicken and Broccoli Stir-fry.

Week 4

	Breakfast	Lunch	Dessert	Dinner
Day 22	Bagel Avocado Toast	Cucumber and Tomato Salad	Low-carb berry chia pudding	Low Carb Zucchini Lasagna
Day 23	Skillet Veggie and Egg Scramble	Black Bean Tacos	Cinnamon baked apples	Veggie Stir-fry with Tofu
Day 24	Low Carb Cottage Cheese Pancakes	Pasta Puttanesca with Beef	Low Carb Chocolate Greek Yogurt Ice Cream	Poached cod with tomato basil sauce
Day 25	Spinach & Egg Scramble with Raspberries	Chicken and Rice Soup	Blackberry Cinnamon Muffins	Sheet-Pan Chicken Fajita Bowls
Day 26	Banana Pancakes	Steamed Asian white fish	Banana Oatmeal Cookies	Chicken and Broccoli Stir-fry
Day 27	Oatmeal with Fruit & Nuts	Baked Chicken with Onions & Leeks	Lemon Blueberry Cupcakes	Spaghetti with Tomato and Basil
Day 28	Apple Walnut Pancakes	Tuna Salad lettuce wraps	Greek Yogurt Berry Popsicles	Mediterranean Chickpea Salad

CHAPTER 4: BREAKFAST DELIGHTS

Spinach & Egg Scramble with Raspberries

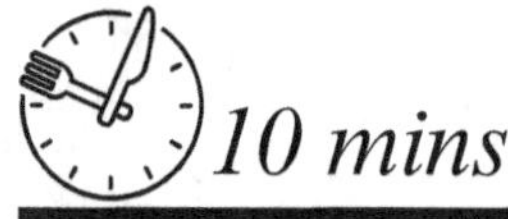 *10 mins*

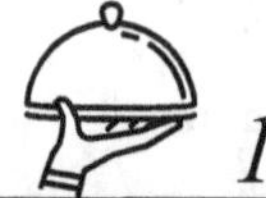 *1*

Prep time   *Cook time*   *Servings*

Ingredients

- 1 teaspoon canola oil
- 1 ½ cups baby spinach (1 1/2 ounces)
- 2 large eggs, lightly beaten
- Pinch of kosher salt
- Pinch of ground pepper
- 1 slice whole-grain bread, toasted
- ½ cup fresh raspberries

Directions

1. In a small nonstick skillet set over medium-high heat, heat the oil. Cook until the spinach is wilted, about 1 to 2 minutes, stirring often. Put the spinach on a platter.
2. Wipe the pan clean, then heat it over medium heat with the eggs. Cook until barely set, 1 to 2 minutes, stirring once or twice to ensure uniform cooking. Combine the spinach, salt, and pepper in a mixing bowl.
3. Serve with toast and raspberries.

Nutrition facts per serving
Calories: 296 | Total Carbohydrate: 21g | Dietary Fiber: 7g | Total Sugars: 5g | Protein: 18g | Total Fat: 16g | Sodium: 394mg

Banana Pancakes

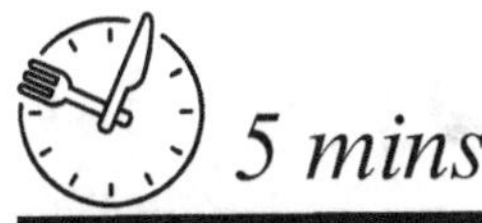 *5 mins*
Prep time

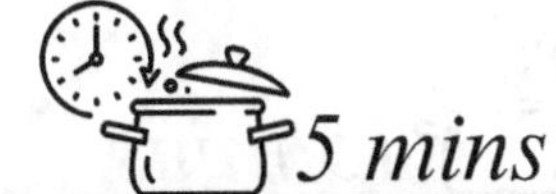 *5 mins*
Cook time

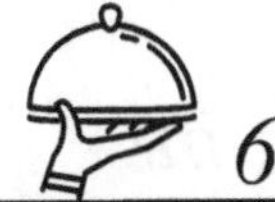 6
Servings

Ingredients

- 1 small banana slightly green to yellow
- 2 large eggs
- ½ tsp butter or coconut oil for cooking

Directions

1. Use a fork to mash the banana.
2. Whisk the eggs together in a mixing bowl. Mix in the mashed banana with the eggs until well combined.
3. Melt the butter or coconut oil in a medium-sized frying pan.
4. 2 tbsp batter per pancake. Cook for 1 minute, or until the bottom of the pancake is slightly browned.
5. Flip the pancake (very gently because the batter is rather moist and the pancakes can easily shatter) then continue to fry the other side.
6. Serve warm with non-fat Greek yogurt, a few tart/sharp berries, nuts, mixed seeds, and, if desired, sweetener or agave nectar.

Nutrition facts per serving
Calories: 42 | Carbohydrates: 4g | Protein: 2g | Fat: 2g | Fiber: 1g | Total sugars: 2g

Blackberry Cinnamon Muffins

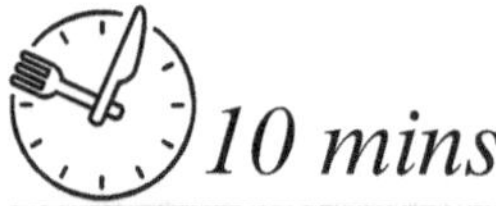 *10 mins*
 *15 mins*
 *12*

Prep time | *Cook time* | *Servings*

Ingredients

- 3/4 cup coconut sugar
- 2 large eggs
- 1/3 cup oil
- 1 cup unsweetened almond milk
- 1 3/4 cups + 2 tablespoons whole wheat white flour
- 1 1/2 teaspoons ground cinnamon
- 1 1/2 teaspoons baking powder
- 1/4 teaspoon baking soda
- 1/4 teaspoon sea salt
- 1 cup blackberries coarsely chopped

Nutrition facts per serving
Calories: 167 | Carbohydrates: 23g | Protein: 4g | Fat: 8g | Sodium: 183mg | Fiber: 3g | Total sugar: 7g

Directions

1. Preheat the oven to 400°F. Line a regular muffin tray with paper liners and coat the liners with cooking spray.
2. In a large mixing basin, whisk together the sugar, eggs, and oil until thoroughly incorporated. Whisk in the milk until smooth.
3. Add the flour to the wet ingredients, then sprinkle with the baking powder, baking soda, cinnamon, and salt.
4. Stir carefully to incorporate the wet and dry ingredients. Fold in the blackberries carefully. Divide the batter evenly among the muffin cups.
5. Bake the muffins for approximately 15 minutes, or until golden brown and a toothpick inserted into the center comes out clean.

34

6. Cool on a wire rack for 10 minutes before removing the muffins from the pan and continuing to cool on the wire rack.

Breakfast Salad with Egg & Salsa Verde Vinaigrette

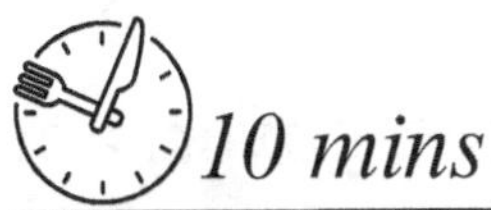 *10 mins*

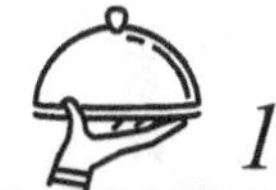 *1*

| *Prep time* | *Cook time* | *Servings* |

Ingredients

- 3 tablespoons salsa verde
- 1 tablespoon+1 tsp. olive oil, divided
- 2 tablespoons chopped cilantro, plus more for garnish
- 2 cups of mesclun or salad greens
- 8 blue corn tortilla chips, broken into large pieces
- ½ cup canned red kidney beans, rinsed
- ¼ avocado, sliced
- 1 large egg

Nutrition facts per serving
Calories: 527 | Total Carbohydrate: 37g | Dietary Fiber: 13g | Total Sugars: 2g | Protein: 16g | Total Fat: 34g | Sodium: 660mg

Directions

1. In a small bowl, combine the salsa, 1 tablespoon oil, and cilantro. In a shallow dinner dish, toss half the mixture with mesclun (or other greens).
2. Top the salad with chips, beans, and avocado.
3. In a small nonstick skillet over medium-high heat, heat the remaining 1 teaspoon of oil.
4. Fry the egg for 2 minutes, or until the white is totally cooked but the yolk is still somewhat runny.
5. Serve the salad with the egg on top. Drizzle with the remaining salsa vinaigrette and, if preferred, top with extra cilantro.

35

Skillet Veggie and Egg Scramble

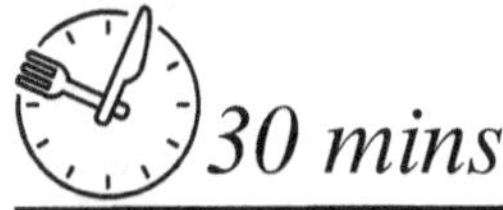 *30 mins*

Prep time

Cook time

 *4*

Servings

Ingredients

- 2 tablespoons olive oil
- 12 ounces baby potatoes, thinly sliced
- 4 cups of thinly sliced vegetables, such as mushrooms, bell peppers, and/or zucchini (14 oz.)
- 3 scallions, thinly sliced, green and white parts separated
- 1 teaspoon minced fresh herbs, such as rosemary or thyme
- 6 large eggs (or 4 large eggs plus 4 egg whites), lightly beaten
- 2 cups of packed leafy greens, such as baby spinach or baby kale (2 oz.)
- ½ teaspoon salt

Nutrition facts per serving
Calories: 254 | Fat: 14g | Carbs: 20g | Protein: 12g | Sodium: 415mg | Total sugars: 5g | Dietary Fiber: 4g

Directions

1. In a large cast-iron or nonstick skillet, heat the oil over medium heat. Add the potatoes, cover, and simmer, turning occasionally, for approximately 8 minutes, or until they start to soften.

2. Add the sliced veggies and scallion whites; simmer uncovered, turning occasionally, for 8 to 10 minutes, or until the vegetables are soft and lightly browned. Add the herbs and stir. Transfer the vegetable mixture to the perimeter of the pan.

3. Turn down the heat to medium-low. Place the eggs and scallions in the middle of the pan. Cook for approximately two minutes, stirring occasionally, or until the eggs are lightly scrambled.

4. Add kale to the eggs and stir. Take off the heat and give everything a good swirl. Add salt and stir.

Apple Walnut Pancakes

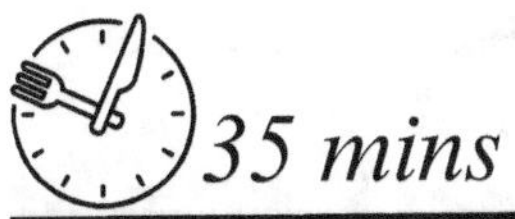 *35 mins*  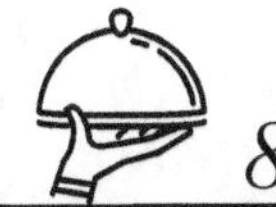 *8*

Prep time | *Cook time* | *Servings*

Ingredients

- 1 cup flour
- 2 ½ teaspoons baking powder
- ½ teaspoon salt
- ½ teaspoon cinnamon
- 1 cup low-fat milk
- 2 teaspoons cooking oil
- 1 egg, beaten
- ½ cup apple, finely chopped
- ¼ cup walnuts, chopped
- 2 tablespoons butter

Directions

1. In a mixing basin, combine the dry ingredients.
2. Mix in the milk, oil, and egg to the dry ingredients.
3. Mix in the chopped apples and walnuts.
4. Melt a tiny quantity of butter on the surface of a hot griddle.
5. When the griddle is hot, pour 1/4 cup batter over it.
6. Cook until little bubbles develop on the surface of the pancake.
7. Peek beneath the pancake to ensure that it seems to be done.
8. Flip to the other side and ensure the pancake is done.
9. Repeat for all the batter.

Nutrition facts per serving
Calories: 142.9 | Total Fat: 7.2g | Sodium: 311.6mg | Total Carbohydrate: 15.7g | Dietary Fiber: 0.9g | Sugars: 1g | Protein: 4.2g

Oatmeal with Fruit & Nuts

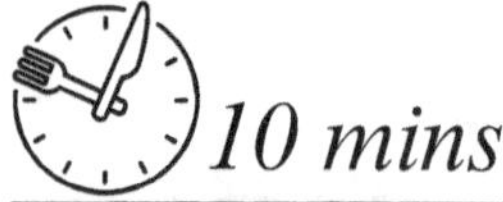 *10 mins*

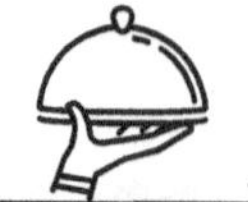 *1*

Prep time **Cook time** **Servings**

Ingredients

- ½ cup old-fashioned oats
- 1 cup low-fat milk
- ¼ cup nonfat plain Greek yogurt
- ¼ cup chopped apple
- 1 tablespoon walnuts, toasted if desired

Directions

1. In a small saucepan, mix the milk and oats. Bring to a boil over high heat, then lower the heat to medium and simmer, stirring constantly, for 4 to 5 minutes, or until the oats are soft and creamy.
2. After turning off the heat, cover and leave for two minutes.
3. Top with yogurt, apples, and walnuts, and serve.

Nutrition facts per serving
Calories: 341 | Total Carbohydrate: 47g | Dietary Fiber: 5g | Total Sugars: 18g | Protein: 22g | Total Fat: 8g | Calcium: 390mg

Bagel Avocado Toast

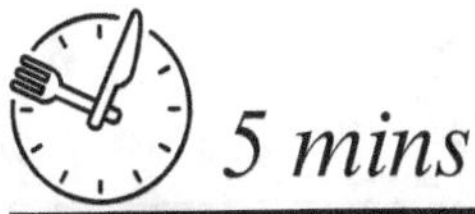 *5 mins*
Prep time

Cook time

 *1*
Servings

Ingredients

- ¼ medium avocado, mashed
- 1 slice whole-grain bread, toasted
- 2 teaspoons bagel seasoning
- Pinch of sea salt

Directions

1. On toast, spread avocado. Season with salt and bagel seasoning to taste.

Nutrition facts per serving
Calories: 172 | Total
Carbohydrate: 18g | Dietary
Fiber: 6g | Total Sugars: 2g |
Added Sugars: 1g | Protein: 5g |
Total Fat: 10g | Sodium: 252mg

Bagel Avocado Toast

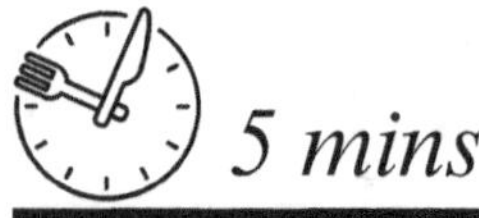 5 mins
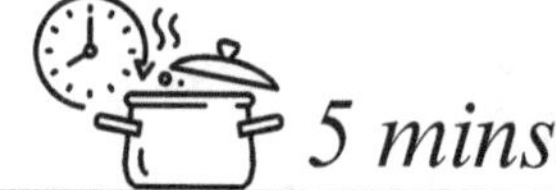 5 mins
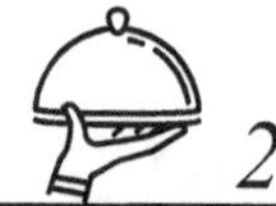 2

| Prep time | Cook time | Servings |

Ingredients

- 3 egg whites approximately 130 grams
- 2½ tablespoons blueberries approximately 1 ounce
- ¼ cup water
- ½ cup rolled oats
- 1 scoop vanilla protein powder
- 1 tablespoon stevia in the raw
- ½ teaspoon baking powder
- cooking spray
- toppings like sugar-free syrup, berries, or chocolate chips (optional)

Nutrition facts per serving
Calories: 182 | Fat: 1.8g |
Sodium: 157mg |
Carbohydrates: 16.6g | Fiber:
2.3g | Sugar: 2.4g| Protein:
22.2g

Directions

1. In a blender, combine the egg whites, water, oats, stevia, vanilla protein powder, and blueberries. Blend it well until smooth.
2. Apply a thin layer of cooking spray to a small skillet and preheat it over medium heat.
3. When the pan is heated, add the pancake batter and tilt it to ensure that the batter covers the whole surface in a uniform layer.
4. Cook each pancake for approximately one minute, or until you notice air bubbles forming on the pancake batter's top and the edges beginning to color. When the pancake is entirely cooked, flip it over and cook for an additional minute.
5. After that, turn off the heat and put it away. Continue doing this until all of the batter has been utilized.

40

6. Garnish with a little amount of sugar-free syrup and present alongside fresh berries. Top with chocolate chips, berries, or sugar-free syrup.

Chocolate Chia Seed Pudding with Almond Milk

 **5 mins**
Prep time

 **1 hr**
Cool time

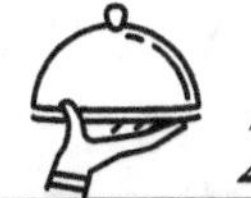 **2**
Servings

Ingredients

- 1/2 cup chia seeds
- 1⅓ cup unsweetened almond milk
- 1/3 cup cocoa powder
- 4 tablespoon Stevia (or sweetener of choice)
- 3/4 teaspoon sea salt

Directions

1. Before combining with the dry ingredients, make sure your cocoa powder is lump-free by sifting it through a sifter.
2. Cocoa powder and sea salt should be combined in a mixing basin. Add the stevia and chia seeds and mix well.
3. Add the almond milk and mix well.
4. Put in a container with a lid and chill for an hour, or better yet, overnight.

Nutrition facts per serving
Calories: 172 | Total
Carbohydrate: 18g | Dietary
Fiber: 6g | Total Sugars: 2g |
Added Sugars: 1g | Protein: 5g |
Total Fat: 10g | Sodium: 252mg

Note: The longer the chia seeds soak in liquid, the more liquid they absorb, producing a smoother pudding.
Chia pudding may be refrigerated in an airtight container for 3–4 days.

Low Carb Cottage Cheese Pancakes

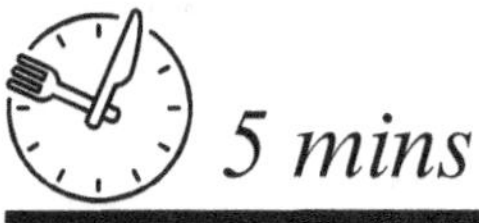 *5 mins*
Prep time

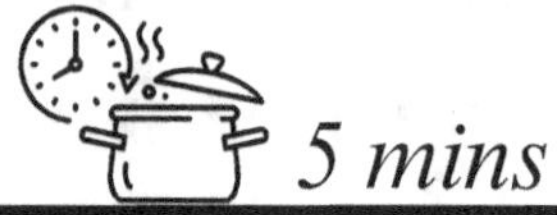 *5 mins*
Cook time

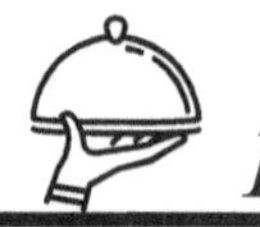 *1*
Servings

Ingredients

- ½ cup low-fat cottage cheese
- ¼ cup oats
- 2 egg Whites
- 1 teaspoon vanilla extract
- 1 tablespoon Stevia in the raw (only if you want the pancakes to be sweet)

Directions

1. Pour the cottage cheese and egg whites into the blender first, then add the oats, vanilla extract, and Tbsp of stevia.
2. Blend the ingredients together until smooth.
3. Spray a pan with cooking spray and set it over medium heat.
4. Add the batter once the pan is hot. Depending on how much batter you add, it will make 1-2 large pancakes or 3 smaller pancakes.
5. Cook each pancake until browned on both sides.
6. Serve with fresh berries, sugar-free jam, or peanut butter.

Nutrition facts per serving
Calories: 205 | Fat: 1.5g |
Sodium: 580mg |
Carbohydrates: 19g | Fiber: 2g |
Sugar: 5.5g | Protein: 24.5g

CHAPTER 5:

DELICIOUS DESSERTS

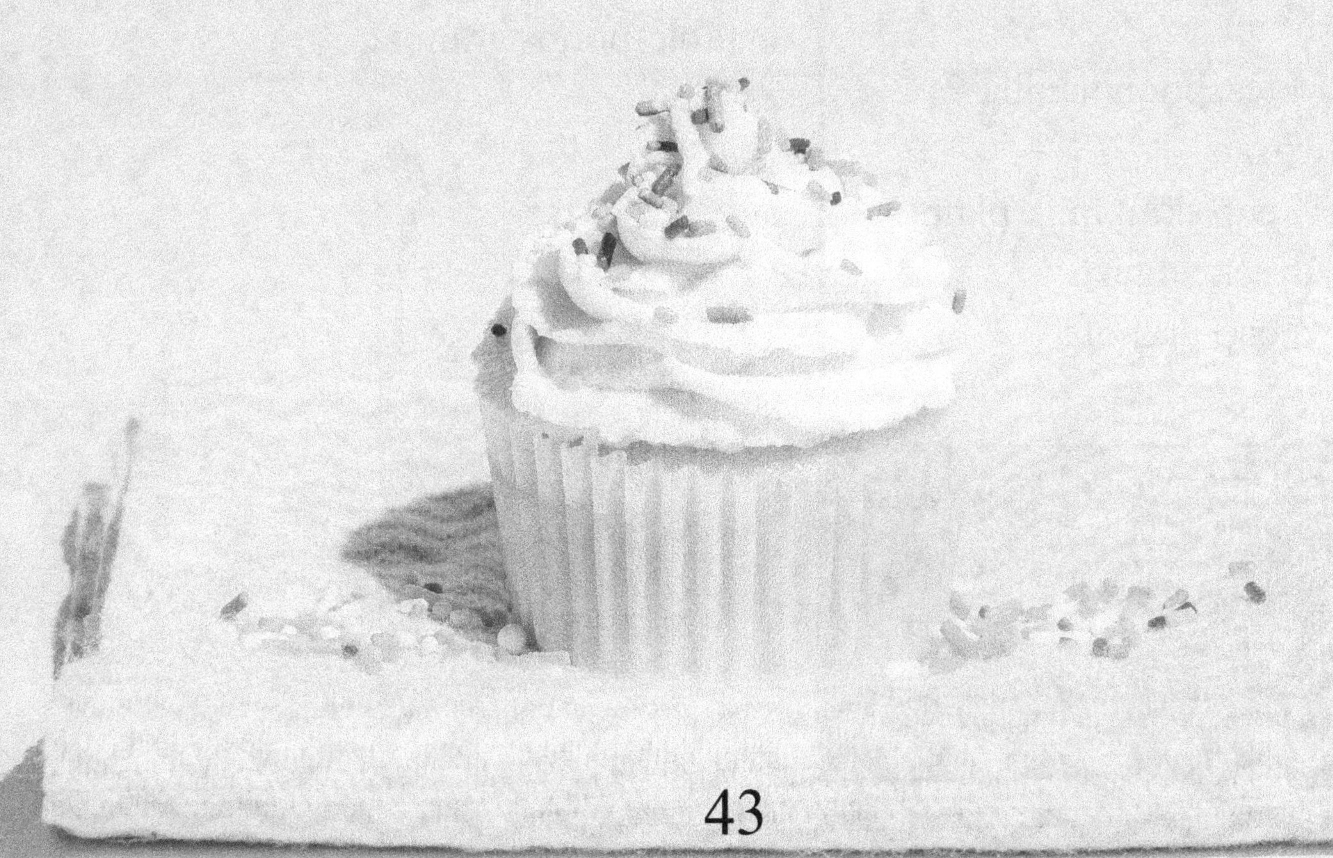

Low-carb berry chia pudding

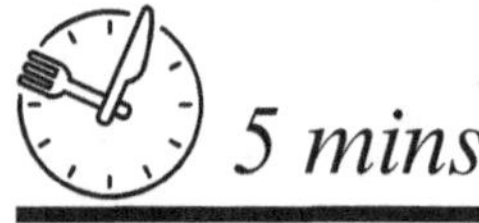 *5 mins*
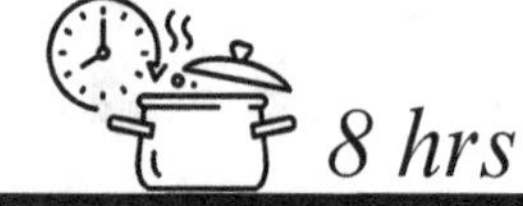 *8 hrs*
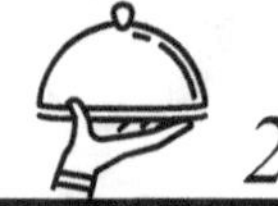 *2*

| *Prep time* | *Additional time* | *Servings* |

Ingredients

- 1¾ cups blackberries, raspberries and/or diced mango (fresh or frozen), divided
- 1 cup unsweetened almond milk or milk of choice
- ¼ cup chia seeds
- 1 tablespoon pure maple syrup
- ¾ teaspoon vanilla extract
- ½ cup skim milk plain Greek yogurt
- ¼ cup granola

Directions

1. In a blender or food processor, puree 1 1/4 cups of fruit and milk until smooth. Scrape into a medium mixing basin; stir in chia, syrup, and vanilla. Refrigerate for at least 8 hours or up to 3 days.
2. Divide the pudding into two dishes and top with 1/4 cup of the leftover fruit, 1/4 cup yogurt, and 2 tablespoons granola.

Nutrition facts per serving
Total Carbohydrate: 39g |
Dietary Fiber: 15g | Total
Sugars: 18g | Added Sugars: 6g |
Protein: 14g | Total Fat: 15g |
Sodium: 125mg

Cinnamon baked apples

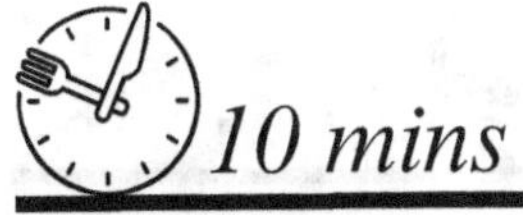 **10 mins**
Prep time

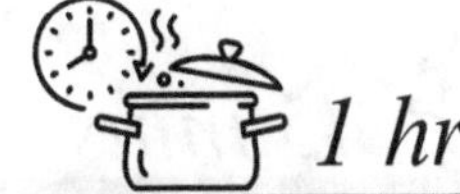 **1 hr**
Cook time

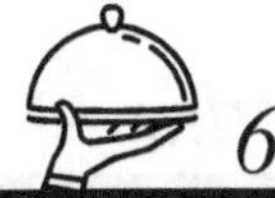 **6**
Servings

Ingredients

- 6-7 medium to large apples
- 2 Tbsp lemon juice
- 1 Tbsp coconut oil (optional)
- 2/3 cup coconut sugar
- 1 ½ tsp ground cinnamon
- 3/4 tsp fresh grated ginger
- 1 pinch nutmeg
- 3 Tbsp cornstarch or arrowroot starch (for thickening the sauce)
- 3 Tbsp fresh apple juice or water
- 1 pinch sea salt
- Coconut Whipped Cream (optional)
- Vanilla Bean Coconut Ice Cream (optional)

Nutrition facts per serving
Calories: 195 | Carbohydrates: 50.6 g | Protein: 0.3 g | Fat: 0.2 g | Sodium: 15 mg | Fiber: 3 g | Sugar: 39.7 g

Directions

1. Preheat the oven to 350°F (176°C) and prepare a 9×13-inch baking dish.
2. Apples should be peeled and cored, quartered, and thinly sliced lengthwise using a paring knife. Just be consistent so they cook evenly.
3. Add to the baking dish and top with lemon juice, coconut oil (optional), coconut sugar, cinnamon, ginger, nutmeg, cornstarch (or arrowroot), apple juice (or water), and a good amount of salt. Toss to mix. Then, lightly wrap with foil.
4. Bake for 45 minutes, covered. Then, gently remove the foil and bake for a further 10-15 minutes, or until the apples are fork soft (particularly in the middle of the dish) and slightly caramelized.
5. Enjoy plain or with Coconut Whipped Cream or Vanilla Bean Coconut Ice Cream! Best when fresh, but leftovers stay covered in the fridge for 3-4 days. Reheat in the microwave or in a 350°F (176°C) oven (covered) until warmed through. If the "caramel" sauce is too thick, thin it up with a little water.

Spiced Pumpkin Cookies

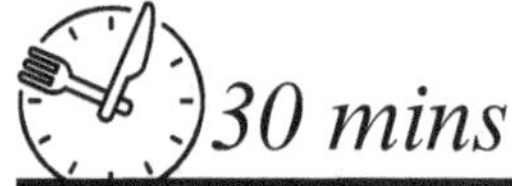 30 mins   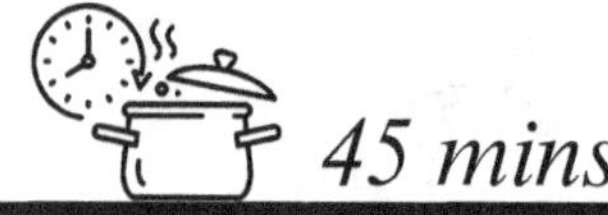 45 mins   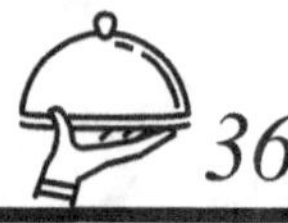 36

Prep time   *Cook time*   *Servings*

Ingredients

- 2/3 cup whole-wheat pastry flour
- 2/3 cup all-purpose flour
- 1 teaspoon baking powder
- ½ teaspoon baking soda
- ½ teaspoon salt
- 1 teaspoon ground cinnamon
- ½ teaspoon ground ginger
- ¼ teaspoon ground allspice
- 1/4 teaspoon freshly grated nutmeg
- 2 large eggs
- 3/4 cup packed light brown sugar or 1/3 cup Splenda Sugar Blend
- 3/4 cup canned unseasoned pumpkin puree
- ¼ cup canola oil
- ¼ cup dark molasses
- 1 cup raisins

Nutrition facts per serving
Calories: 72 | Total Carbohydrate: 13g | Dietary Fiber: 1g | Total Sugars: 9g | Added Sugars: 7g | Protein: 1g | Total Fat: 2g | Sodium: 70mg

Directions

1. Preheat the oven to 350°F. Spray three baking sheets with nonstick cooking spray.

2. In a large mixing bowl, combine the whole-wheat flour, all-purpose flour, baking powder, baking soda, salt, cinnamon, ginger, allspice, and nutmeg.

3. In a separate bowl, whisk together the eggs, brown sugar (or Splenda), pumpkin, oil, and molasses. Stir in the dry ingredients and raisins until fully incorporated.

4. Drop the batter onto the prepared baking sheets by level tablespoonfuls, placing the cookies 1 1/2 inches apart.

5. Bake the cookies for 10 to 12 minutes, or until firm to the touch and faintly brown on top, swapping the pans back and forth halfway through. Allow to cool on a wire rack.

46

Plan ahead of time Tip: For up to 2 days, store cookies in an airtight container with wax paper between the layers, or freeze for extended storage.

Strawberry-Mango Nice Cream

 5 mins
Prep time

Cook time

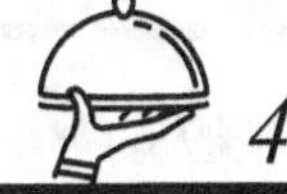 4
Servings

Ingredients

- 12 ounces frozen mango chunks
- 8 ounces frozen sliced strawberries
- 1 tablespoon lime juice

Directions

1. In a food processor, combine mango, strawberries, and lime juice; process for 1–2 minutes. Scrape down the sides of the processor.
2. Continue processing for another 2 to 3 minutes, or until smooth, adding up to 1/2 cup water as needed to assist the fruit process.

Nutrition facts per serving
Serving Size 3/4 cup
Calories: 70 | Total
Carbohydrate: 17g | Dietary
Fiber: 3g | Total Sugars: 14g |
Protein: 1g | Total Fat: 1g |
Sodium: 2mg

Greek Yogurt Berry Popsicles

 *2 hrs*

Prep time

Cook time

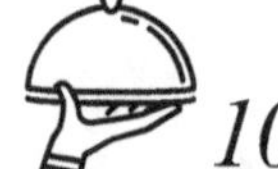 *10*

Servings

Ingredients

- 2 cups low fat vanilla Greek yogurt
- 2 cups nonfat milk
- 2 cups mixed berries (fresh or frozen)
- 1 banana
- 1 teaspoon cinnamon

Directions

1. In a high-speed blender, purée all of the ingredients until smooth.
2. Pour contents into popsicle molds, put in popsicle sticks, and freeze until firm.

Nutrition facts per serving
Calories: 99 | Carbohydrates: 15.3g | Protein: 5.5g | Fat: 2.4g | Sodium: 47mg | Fiber: 1g | Sugar: 12.3g

Sugar-free Coconut Macaroons

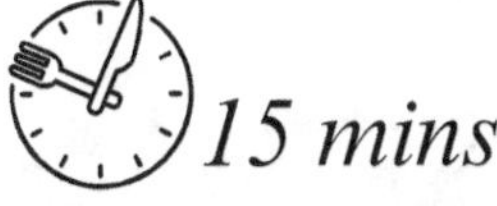 *15 mins*  *32 mins* 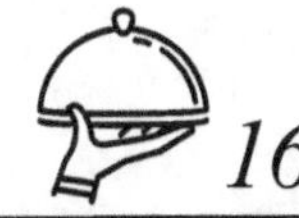 *16*

Prep time | *Cook time* | *Servings*

Ingredients

- 2/3 cup slivered almonds
- 1 1/4 cup shredded unsweetened coconut
- 1/3 cup + 3 T Golden Monkfruit Sweetener (see notes)
- generous pinch of salt
- 1/4 cup low-fat Greek Yogurt
- 2 egg whites
- 2 tsp. vanilla essence

Nutrition facts per serving
Calories: 75 | Total Fat: 6g |
Sodium: 19mg | Carbohydrates:
3g | Fiber: 2g | Sugar: 1g |
Protein: 2g

Directions

1. Set oven temperature to 325°F/170°C.
2. Using a silicone baking mat or parchment paper, line a baking sheet.
3. Grind the almonds in a small food processor or with the immersion blender's bowl attachment until they are a little chunky but still ground.
4. In a medium-sized dish, combine the crushed almonds, shredded coconut, sugar, and salt; stir with a spoon.
5. To obtain two egg whites, separate two eggs. (Reserve the yolks for another use or throw them away.)
6. To the dry mixture, add the egg whites, Greek yogurt, and vanilla essence. Using a spoon, stir the ingredients until thoroughly blended.
7. One spoonful of dough at a time, scoop out, shape into a ball, and arrange approximately 2 inches apart on the baking sheet.
8. Press each ball into a cookie that is just about 1/2 inch thick using a fork. Due to the crumbly nature of the batter, you can also use the fork to push the edges together.
9. Bake for 30 to 32 minutes, or until cookies are firm and beginning to color attractively around the edges.

49

Lemon Blueberry Cupcakes

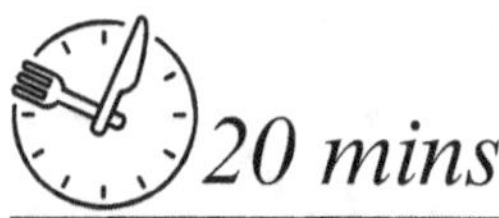 **20 mins**

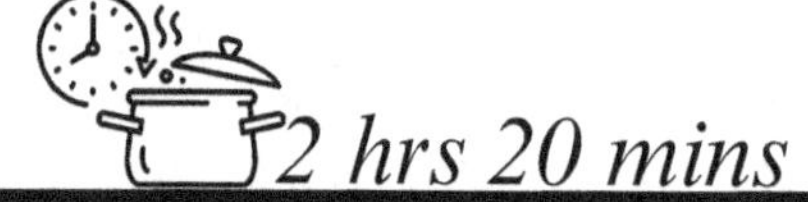 **2 hrs 20 mins**

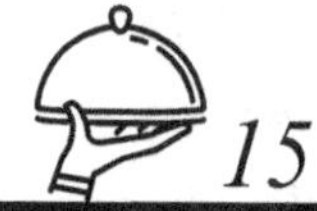 **15**

Prep time | Cook time | Servings

Ingredients

- 1 and 1/2 cups (188g) all-purpose flour (spooned & leveled)
- 2 teaspoons baking powder
- 1/2 teaspoon salt
- 1/2 cup (8 Tbsp; 113g) unsalted butter, softened to room temperature
- 1 cup (200g) granulated sugar
- 1 Tablespoon lemon zest
- 2 large eggs, at room temperature
- 1 and 1/2 teaspoons pure vanilla extract
- 1/2 cup (120ml) whole milk or buttermilk, at room temperature
- 1/4 cup (60ml) fresh lemon juice
- 1 cup (140g) fresh or frozen blueberries, tossed in 1 Tablespoon flour

Directions

1. Preheat the oven to 350°F/177°C. Make a 12-cup muffin pan with cupcake liners.

2. In a large mixing basin, sift the flour, baking powder, and salt together. Put aside.

3. In a large mixing basin, cream together the butter, sugar, and lemon zest using a hand mixer or stand mixer on medium-high speed for 2 minutes. Scrape the sides and bottom of the bowl as required.

4. Add eggs and vanilla extract and beat on medium-high speed for 1 minute, or until blended. Scrape the sides and bottom of the bowl as required. Mix in the dry ingredients first, then gently pour in the milk and lemon juice. Beat till just blended. Mix in the floured blueberries. Don't overmix.

Cream Cheese Frosting:

- 8 ounces (226g) full-fat brick cream cheese, softened to room temperature
- 1/4 cup (4 Tbsp; 56g) unsalted butter, softened to room temperature
- 2 cups (240g) confectioners' sugar
- 1 teaspoon pure vanilla extract
- pinch salt
- optional: lemon slices and extra blueberries for garnish

Nutrition facts per serving
Calories: 315 | Total Fat: 16g | Sodium: 280mg | Total Carbohydrates: 39g | Dietary Fiber: 1g | Sugars: 26g | Protein: 3g

5. Fill the liners only 2/3 full to avoid batter pouring over the sides. Bake for 18-21 minutes, or until a toothpick inserted in the center comes out clean. Bake for 11-13 minutes at the same oven temperature for about 30-36 small cupcakes. Allow the cupcakes to cool fully before icing them.

6. To make the frosting: In a large mixing basin, beat the cream cheese and butter on medium speed with a hand mixer or stand mixer fitted with a whisk or paddle attachment until smooth, about 2 minutes.

7. Add the confectioners' sugar, vanilla extract, salt and beat on low for 30 seconds, then increase to medium-high speed and beat for 2 minutes. If preferred, add an extra pinch of salt. If you intend to frost piping designs with this frosting, chill it for at least 20 minutes first.

8. Top cooled cupcakes with optional topping, if desired. Refrigerate frosted cupcakes uncovered for at least 20 minutes before serving to help set the icing.

9. Refrigerate any leftover cupcakes for up to 5 days. A cupcake carrier facilitates storage and transportation.

Banana Oatmeal Cookies

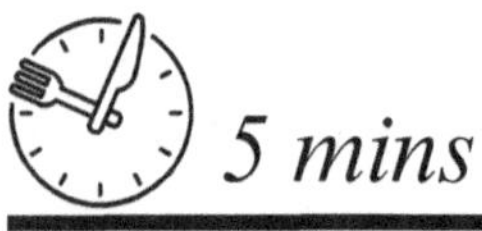 *5 mins*
Prep time

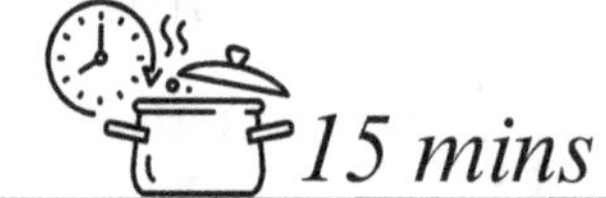 *15 mins*
Cook time

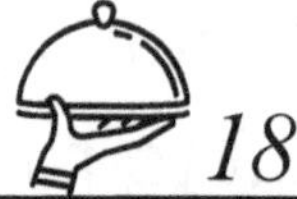 *18*
Servings

Ingredients

- 3 bananas overripe (about 1 ¼ cups mashed banana)
- 2 Tbsp honey (or maple syrup)
- 1 egg
- 1 tsp pure vanilla extract
- 1 ½ cup quick cooking oats
- 1 tsp ground cinnamon
- ¼ tsp fine sea salt
- ½ cup chocolate chips or other add-ins like shredded coconut, dried cranberries, raisins, etc.

Nutrition facts per serving
Calories: 79 | Carbohydrates: 15g | Protein: 2g | Fat: 2g | Sodium: 40mg | Fiber: 1g | Sugar: 8g

Directions

1. Preheat the oven to 350°F. Set aside two baking sheets lined with parchment paper.
2. Mash the bananas in a large mixing dish.
3. Stir in the honey, egg, and vanilla extract.
4. Stir in the oats, cinnamon, and sea salt until well blended.
5. If preferred, use a whisk to mix until equally distributed.
6. Measure out chunks of dough using a 1 tablespoon measuring spoon or a 12 tablespoon cookie scoop and lay them approximately 2" apart on the prepared baking sheet.
7. Bake for 12–15 minutes, or until the tops are just set and the bottoms are gently browned, in a preheated oven.
8. Allow to cool for 5 minutes on the baking sheet before transferring to a wire cooling rack to cool fully.
9. Serve at room temperature or slightly heated.

52

Coconut Milk Shake

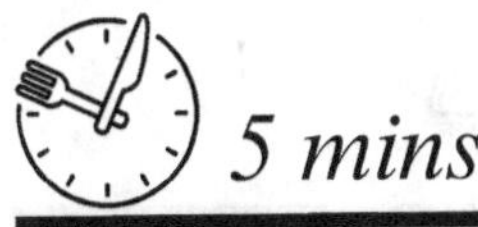 *5 mins*
Prep time

Cook time

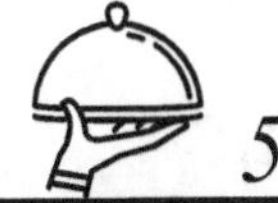 *5*
Servings

Ingredients

- 1 can full-fat coconut milk
- ¼ cup unsweetened almond milk
- ¼ cup unsweetened shredded coconut
- 1 tablespoon chia seeds
- ¼ teaspoon vanilla extract
- 1-2 tablespoon low carb sweetener such as stevia or erythritol

Directions

1. Blend together the coconut milk, almond milk, shredded coconut, chia seeds, vanilla essence, and sweetener in a blender.
2. Blend until the shake is thick and foamy, then add the ice cubes.
3. Pour into a glass and serve. Top with whipped coconut cream and sprinkle with toasted shredded coconut, if desired.

Nutrition facts per serving
Calories: 220 | Carbohydrates: 10g | Protein: 10g | Fat: 16g | Fiber: 6g | Sugar: 2g

Low Carb Chocolate Greek Yogurt Ice Cream

 *2 hrs*

Prep time

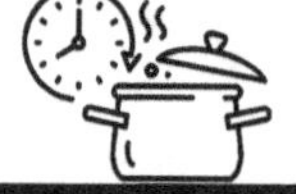

Cook time

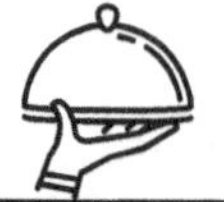 *1*

Servings

Ingredients

- 2½ oz. fat-free Greek yogurt
- ½ oz. vanilla protein powder
- 1 teaspoon unsweetened cocoa powder
- ½ cup unsweetened almond milk
- 1 teaspoon vanilla extract
- 2 tablespoon Stevia to taste
- Almonds & berries (optional)

Nutrition facts per serving
Calories: 127 | Fat: 2.2g |
Sodium: 150mg |
Carbohydrates: 8.1g | Fiber:
2.5g | Sugar: 4.4g | Protein:
20.1g

Directions

1. Thoroughly combine yogurt, protein powder, chocolate, stevia, and almond milk.
2. Place in the freezer or ice cream maker.
3. If making in the freezer, remove the ice cream after an hour and gently flip it over with a spoon to prevent it from forming one giant ice block. Repeat every 30 minutes until the ice cream is the desired consistency (approximately 2 hours total).
4. When you're ready to serve, take the ice cream out of the freezer 5-10 minutes before serving to allow it to soften somewhat.

DAILY FOOD JOURNAL

DATE:

BREAKFAST	LUNCH	DESSERT	DINNER

TODAY'S WORKOUT

WATER INTAKE

NOTES

DAILY FOOD JOURNAL

DATE:

BREAKFAST	LUNCH	DESSERT	DINNER

TODAY'S WORKOUT

WATER INTAKE

NOTES

DAILY FOOD JOURNAL

DATE:

BREAKFAST	LUNCH	DESSERT	DINNER

TODAY'S WORKOUT

WATER INTAKE

NOTES

DAILY FOOD JOURNAL

DATE:

BREAKFAST	LUNCH	DESSERT	DINNER

TODAY'S WORKOUT

WATER INTAKE

NOTES

DAILY FOOD JOURNAL

DATE:

BREAKFAST	LUNCH	DESSERT	DINNER

TODAY'S WORKOUT

WATER INTAKE

NOTES

DAILY FOOD JOURNAL

DATE:

BREAKFAST	LUNCH	DESSERT	DINNER

TODAY'S WORKOUT

WATER INTAKE

NOTES

DAILY FOOD JOURNAL

DATE:

BREAKFAST	LUNCH	DESSERT	DINNER

TODAY'S WORKOUT

WATER INTAKE

NOTES

WEEKLY PLANNER

WEEK :

MONDAY

- ☐ _______________________
- ☐ _______________________
- ☐ _______________________
- ☐ _______________________

TUESDAY

- ☐ _______________________
- ☐ _______________________
- ☐ _______________________
- ☐ _______________________

WEDNESDAY

- ☐ _______________________
- ☐ _______________________
- ☐ _______________________
- ☐ _______________________

THURSDAY

- ☐ _______________________
- ☐ _______________________
- ☐ _______________________
- ☐ _______________________

FRIDAY

- ☐ _______________________
- ☐ _______________________
- ☐ _______________________
- ☐ _______________________

SATURDAY

- ☐ _______________________
- ☐ _______________________
- ☐ _______________________
- ☐ _______________________

SUNDAY

- ☐ _______________________
- ☐ _______________________
- ☐ _______________________
- ☐ _______________________

NOTE :

Chapter 6
Sensational Salads

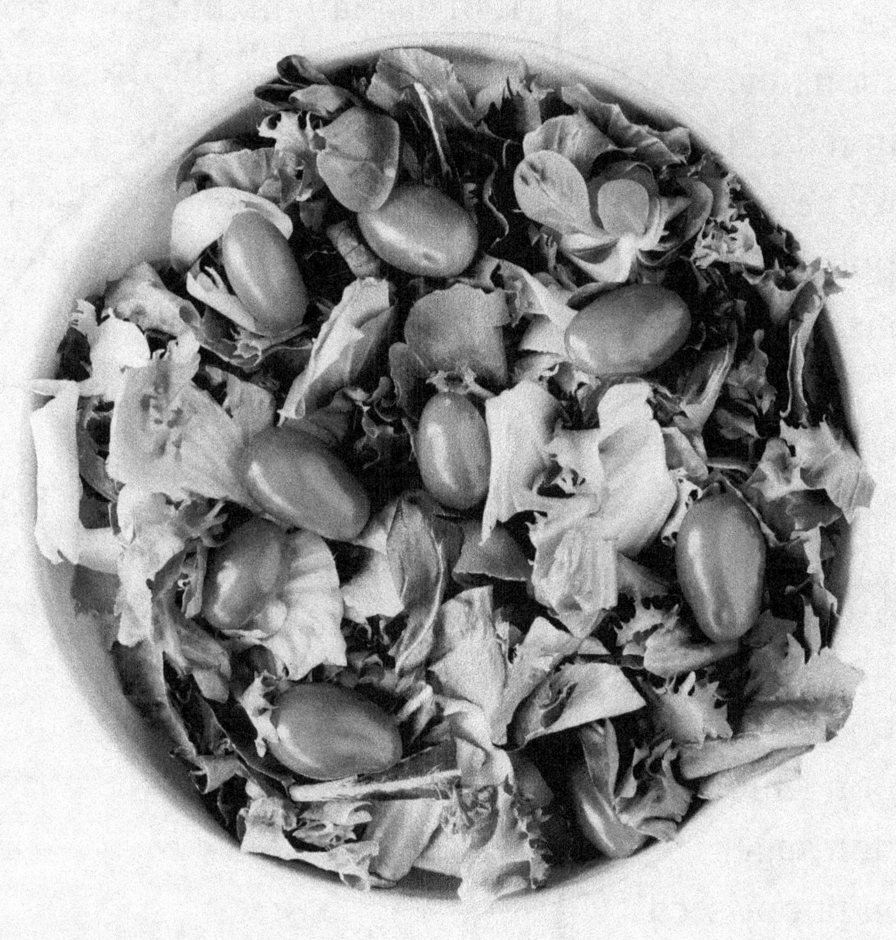

Broccoli and Cranberry Salad

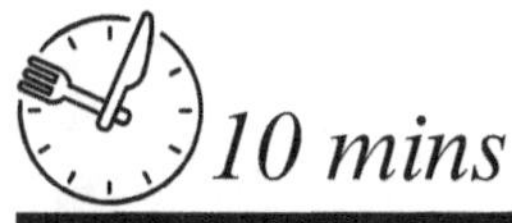 *10 mins*
Prep time

Cook time

 *12*
Servings

Ingredients

- 8 cups broccoli washed and chopped
- 4 green onions sliced (or 1/4 cup red onion)
- ½ cup dried cranberries
- 1 green apple diced
- 2 teaspoons fresh lemon juice
- ⅓ cup pecans chopped, optional

DRESSING:
- 1 cup mayonnaise
- ⅓ cup sour cream
- 1 tablespoon cider vinegar
- 1 tablespoon lemon juice
- 1 tablespoon sugar
- 1 teaspoon poppy seeds
- Salt & pepper to taste

Nutrition facts per serving
Calories: 211 | Carbohydrates: 12g | Protein: 2g | Fat: 17g | Sodium: 144mg | Fiber: 2g | Sugar: 7g

Directions

1. In a small mixing bowl, combine together all of the dressing ingredients and mix.
2. Toss the apple with 2 teaspoons lemon juice. Place in a large mixing bowl with the remaining ingredients. Toss with the dressing until well combined.
3. Allow at least one hour before serving to chill.

Spinach and Berry Salad

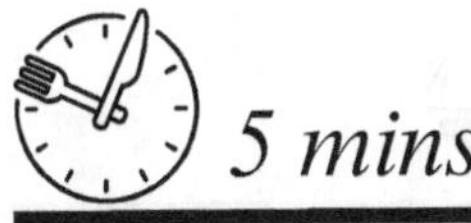 *5 mins*

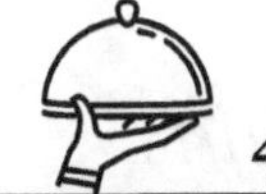 *4*

Prep time | **Cook time** | **Servings**

Ingredients

- 6 cups baby spinach
- 1 cup strawberries, halved
- 1/2 cup raspberries
- 1/2 cup blueberries
- 1/3 cup goat cheese, crumbled
- 1/3 cup red onion, thinly sliced
- 1/4 cup pecans, roughly chopped
- 1/2 recipe Raspberry Vinaigrette

Directions

1. In a large mixing bowl, add the spinach, pecans, red onion, blueberries, raspberries, and goat cheese. Toss to combine.
2. Drizzle the raspberry vinaigrette dressing over the salad.

Nutrition facts per serving
Calories: 283 | Carbs: 16.7g |
Protein: 10.2g | Fat: 20.6g |
Sodium: 295mg | Fiber: 7.2g |
Sugar: 6.2g

Roasted Vegetable Salad

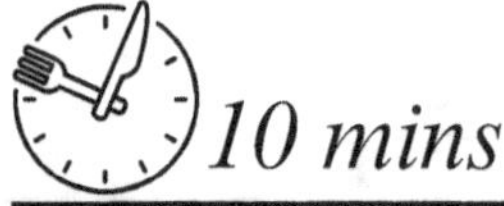 10 mins
 30 mins
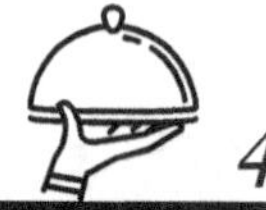 4

Prep time   **Cook time**   **Servings**

Ingredients

- 1 large head of Romaine Lettuce, root trimmed then chopped
- 2 medium Peppers, cored & diced into large chunks
- 2 small Red Onions, peeled & quartered
- 1 medium Eggplant, diced into chunks slightly smaller than the peppers
- 1 medium Zucchini diced into chunks
- 1 medium Sweet Potato, peeled & diced
- 50g crumbled Feta, or more to preference
- 2-3 tbsp Pine Nuts, or to preference
- 1.5 tbsp Olive Oil
- 1/2 tsp each: Oregano, Garlic Powder, Salt
- 1/4 tsp Black Pepper

Directions

1. Dressing: In a jar, combine extra virgin olive oil, balsamic vinegar, honey, dijon mustard, garlic powder, salt, and pepper. Tightly screw on the top and shake until well combined. This may also be done in a small bowl with a whisk. Set to one side.

2. On a large baking sheet, arrange the zucchini, eggplant, peppers, sweet potato, and onions. If there isn't enough room, use two trays; otherwise, the vegetables will steam and get mushy. Mix in the olive oil, oregano, garlic powder, and salt with your hands until equally blended.

3. Roast at 220°C/425°F for 25-35 minutes, or until faintly browned and fork tender, turning once throughout cooking. Remove the dish from the oven and top with pine nuts and feta.

DRESSING

- 1/4 cup Extra Virgin Olive Oil
- 2 tbsp Balsamic Vinegar
- 1 tbsp Honey
- 1 tsp Dijon Mustard
- 1/2 tsp Garlic Powder
- Salt & Pepper, to taste

4. Return to the oven for a few minutes, or until the pine nuts begin to brown and the feta becomes soft and gooey. Allow the vegetables to steam and cool for 5-10 minutes.

5. Salad: Arrange the leaves in a large serving dish, then pour over the vegetables. Drizzle dressing over salad, then toss until evenly incorporated. Serve immediately and enjoy!

Nutrition facts per serving
Calories: 311 | Fat: 20.81g |
Sodium: 131mg |
Carbohydrates: 28.58g | Fiber:
8.9g | Sugar: 16.24g | Protein:
6.42g

Greek Salmon Salad with Tahini Yogurt Dressing

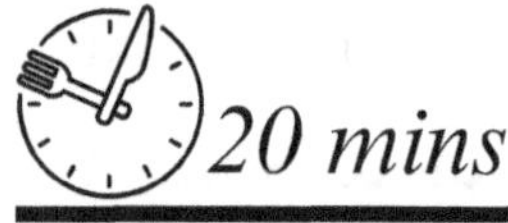 20 mins
Prep time

 10 mins
Cook time

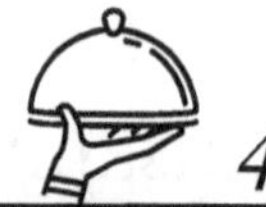 4
Servings

Ingredients

Salmon

- 4 (4 oz) skin-on wild caught salmon fillets
- 1/2 teaspoon dried dill
- 1/2 teaspoon dried oregano
- 1/4 teaspoon granulated garlic
- Kosher salt and fresh ground black pepper to taste

Tahini Yogurt Dressing

- 1/2 cup plain non-fat Greek yogurt
- 1 tablespoon tahini
- 1 1/2 teaspoons olive oil
- 1 lemon, juiced
- 1/4 teaspoon ground cumin
- 1/4 teaspoon dried dill
- 1/4 teaspoon granulated garlic
- 1/4 teaspoon coriander
- Kosher salt and fresh ground black pepper to taste

Directions

1. Preheat the grill over medium-high heat and brush the grill grates with oil. While the grill is heating up, mix all of the salmon spices and smash them with a mortar and pestle or your palms. Evenly sprinkle over the salmon.

2. Place the salmon on the grill, flesh side down, and cook for 3-5 minutes each side, depending on thickness. Remove the grill and let it sit for a few minutes before removing the skin and peeling it apart with a fork.

3. In a small mixing bowl, whisk together all of the dressing ingredients until smooth. Season to taste, then chill until ready to serve.

- 6 cups chopped romaine lettuce
- 1/3 cup thinly sliced red onion
- 1/3 cup kalamata olives
- 2 ounces feta cheese, cubed
- 1 cup diced cucumber
- 1/2 cup cherry tomatoes, halved
- 1 teaspoon olive oil
- 1 teaspoon red wine vinegar
- 1/4 teaspoon dried oregano
- 1/4 teaspoon dried dill
- Kosher salt and fresh ground black pepper to taste

4. Whisk together the red wine vinegar, olive oil, oregano, dill, salt, and pepper in a medium mixing bowl. Combine the chopped cucumber, cherry tomatoes, and red onion in a mixing bowl. To mix, toss everything together.

5. Place the romaine lettuce on a big plate or in a serving dish. Place the leaves on a plate and top with the cucumber combination, olives, feta, and salmon. Dressing should be served on the side.

Nutrition facts per serving
Calories: 361 | Total fat: 21g |
Sodium: 182mg | Carbs: 11g |
Fiber: 3g | Sugar: 5g | Protein: 33g

Cucumber and Tomato Salad

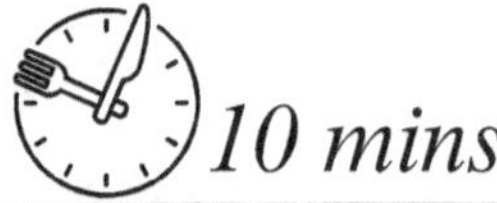 *10 mins*

Prep time

Cook time

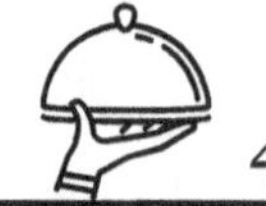 *4*

Servings

Ingredients

- 1 long cucumber, sliced
- 2-3 large tomatoes diced
- ½ red onion sliced
- 1 tablespoon fresh herbs parsley, basil and/or dill, optional
- 2 tablespoons olive oil
- 1 tablespoon red wine vinegar
- Salt & pepper to taste

Directions

1. Toss together all of the ingredients in a mixing basin and mix.
2. Refrigerate for at least 20 minutes before serving.

Nutrition facts per serving
Calories: 104 | Carbohydrates: 7g | Protein: 2g | Fat: 8g | Sodium: 6mg | Fiber: 2g | Sugar: 4g

Spinach and Chickpea Salad

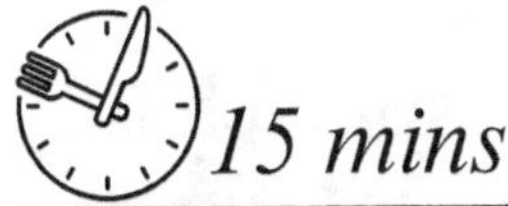 *15 mins*
Prep time

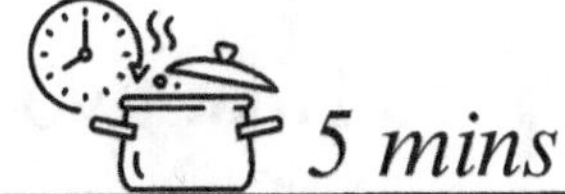 *5 mins*
Cook time

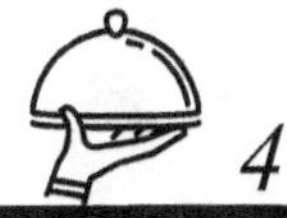 *4*
Servings

Ingredients

For the salad

- 2½ cups canned chickpeas 400 grams (drained)
- 2 cups fresh spinach 100 grams
- 2 shallots
- 10 cherry tomatoes
- 1 tsp sweet smoked paprika 2.30 grams
- 1/2 tsp ground cumin 1.25 grams
- 1 tbsp extra virgin olive oil 15 ml
- pinch sea salt
- dash black pepper

For the sherry vinaigrette

- 2 tbsp extra virgin olive oil 30 ml
- 1/2 tbsp sherry vinegar 8 ml
- 1 clove garlic
- 1 tbsp finely chopped parsley 4 grams
- pinch sea salt
- dash black pepper

Directions

1. Over medium heat, preheat a large nonstick frypan.

2. The canned chickpeas should be drained into a sieve, rinsed under cold water, and shaken off any excess water. Then, add the chickpeas to the heated pan, stirring every minute or so to ensure they are all in a single layer.

3. After 4 minutes, add 1 tablespoon extra virgin olive oil, 1 teaspoon sweet smoked paprika, 1/2 teaspoon ground cumin, and season with sea salt and black pepper. Mix well, remove from the heat, and set aside to cool.

4. Prepare the sherry vinaigrette in the meantime by adding 2 tablespoons extra virgin olive oil, 1/2 tablespoon sherry vinegar, 1 clove of finely grated garlic, 1 tablespoon minced fresh parsley, and a dash of sea salt and black pepper to a small dish.

71

Whisk everything together and set aside.

5. Take two cups of fresh spinach (if not using bagged, wash and pat dry), roughly chop, and add to a big dish.

6. Slice two shallots thinly and cut ten cherry tomatoes in half. Add both to the bowl with the spinach and season with a little sea salt and black pepper. Add the chilled spicy chickpeas and stir everything until thoroughly combined.

7. After transferring the salad to a large serving dish and dressing it with vinaigrette, you can serve it cold or at room temperature. Enjoy!

Nutrition facts per serving
Calories: 400 | Total Fat: 22g |
Sodium: 420mg | Total
Carbohydrates: 50g | Dietary
Fiber: 14g | Sugars: 7g | Protein:
17g

Roasted beet and orange salad

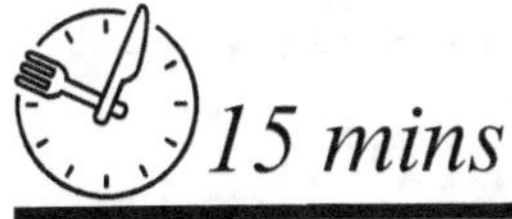 *15 mins*

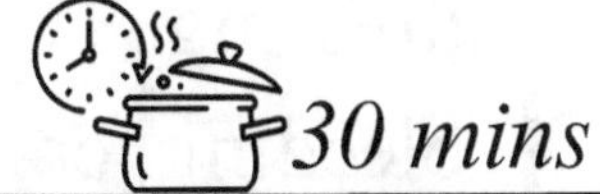 *30 mins*

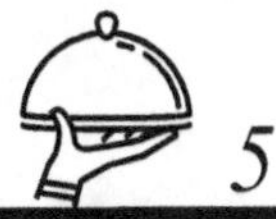 *5*

Prep time   **Cook time**   **Servings**

Ingredients

For the beets:
- 6 medium sized beets, red and yellow
- 2 tablespoons extra virgin olive oil
- 3 heaping cups arugula
- 3 oranges, peeled and cut into wedges
- ½ cup walnuts
- ½ cup goat cheese crumbles

For the beet salad dressing:
- 3 tablespoons fresh orange juice
- ¼ cup extra virgin olive oil
- 2 tablespoons white balsamic vinegar
- 1 tablespoon honey
- Salt and pepper, to taste

Directions

1. Preheat the oven to 400°F. With a vegetable peeler, peel the beets and cut them into two-inch pieces. Two sheets of aluminum foil should be used to line a baking pan. Place the red beets in the center of one sheet of foil and the yellow beets in the center of the other.

2. Drizzle a tablespoon of olive oil over each beet sheet. Fold up the edges and squeeze together to make two pouches. (made two separate pouches so that the colors won't bleed). Place on a baking sheet. Bake for 30 minutes, or until the potatoes are soft.

3. While the beets are roasting, mix together the orange juice, olive oil, white balsamic vinegar, and honey to make the dressing.

4. When the beets are done roasting, combine them with half of the salad dressing. To keep the colors from bleeding, combine them in two separate bowls.

5. On a plate or dish, layer arugula, then top with beets, orange slices, walnuts, and goat cheese. As desired, drizzle with the leftover dressing. Season to taste with salt and pepper. Enjoy!

Nutrition facts per serving
Calories: 384 | Carbs: 26g |
Protein: 8g | Fat: 29g | Sodium:
163mg | Fiber: 5g | Sugar: 18g

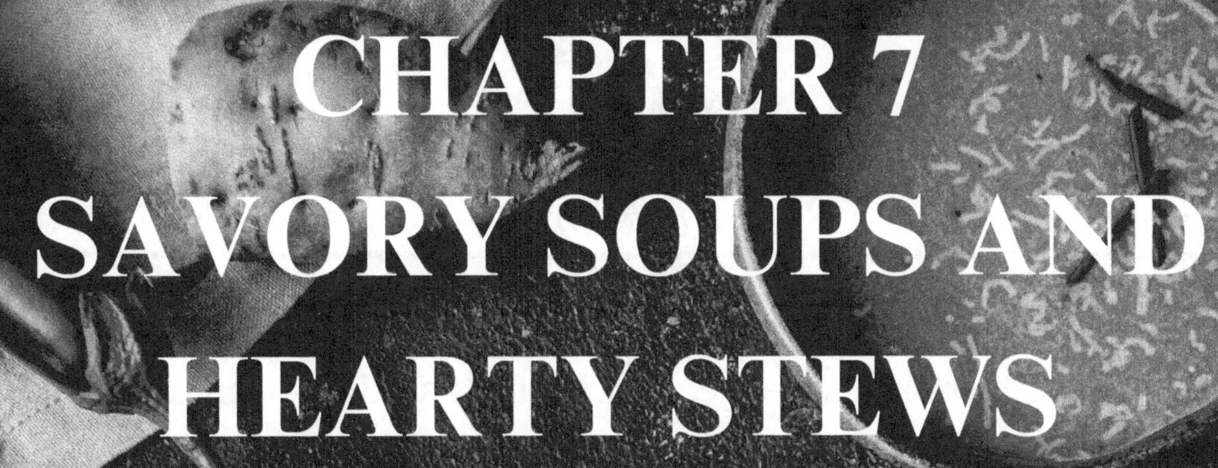

CHAPTER 7
SAVORY SOUPS AND HEARTY STEWS

Cabbage and Sausage Soup

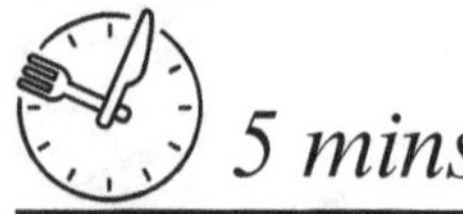 5 mins
 20 mins
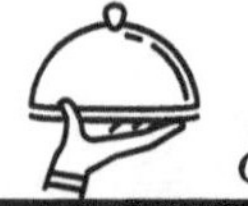 8

| Prep time | Cook time | Servings |

Ingredients

- 16 ounce smoked sausage, sliced
- 1 tablespoon minced garlic
- 1/2 cup onion, chopped
- 1 cup celery, chopped
- 1 cup bell pepper, chopped
- 3/4 cup carrots, chopped
- 3-4 cups cabbage, chopped
- 32 ounces broth (vegetable, beef or chicken)
- 2 teaspoons each onion and garlic powder
- 1 teaspoon each paprika and oregano

Nutrition facts per serving
Calories: 206 | Total fat: 15.2g |
Sodium: 482mg | Carbs: 7.7g |
Fiber: 2.2g | Sugar: 3.6g |
Protein: 9.4g

Directions

1. Preheat a dutch oven or big saucepan over medium heat. Add the sliced sausage to the skillet and cook, turning repeatedly, until browned. (Optional: If you want to remove some of the oil from the skillet, use paper towels to blot the sausage and remove as much oil as required.)
2. Add the garlic, onion, celery, bell pepper, and carrots. Cook for 4-5 minutes, stirring constantly.
3. Stir in the broth, cabbage, and seasonings. Allow the soup to simmer (but not boil) for 10-15 minutes.
4. To taste, season with salt and pepper. Serve immediately.

Mexican Beef Stew

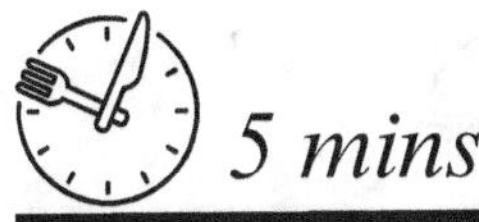 *5 mins*
Prep time

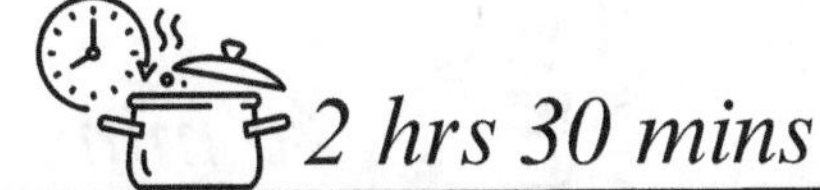 *2 hrs 30 mins*
Cook time

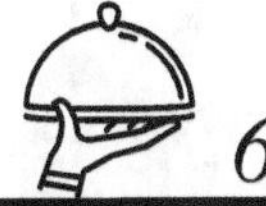 *6*
Servings

Ingredients

- 2 ½ lbs chuck roast, trimmed of fat and cut in bite-sized pieces
- 4 tablespoons flour
- 2 tablespoons olive oil
- 1 large onion, chopped
- 2 cloves garlic, chopped
- 2 -3 jalapeno peppers, seeded and minced
- 3 cups beef stock
- 2 tablespoons tomato paste
- 4 teaspoons cumin
- 1 teaspoon chili powder

Directions

1. Heat the oven to 350 degrees Fahrenheit.
2. Coat the meat pieces in flour and fry them quickly in oil in a Dutch oven.
3. Bring the beef stock, tomato paste, onion, garlic, jalapeño, cumin, and chili powder to a simmer over the cooker.
4. When the beef is very soft, bake it in a Dutch oven, covered, for two to two and a half hours.
5. Serve heated, folded into tortillas, or over rice.

Nutrition facts per serving
Calories: 355.5 | Total Fat: 16.7 g | Sodium: 653 mg | Total Carbohydrate: 9.4 g | Dietary Fiber: 1.2 g | Sugars: 2 g | Protein: 42.8 g

Quinoa and Vegetable Soup

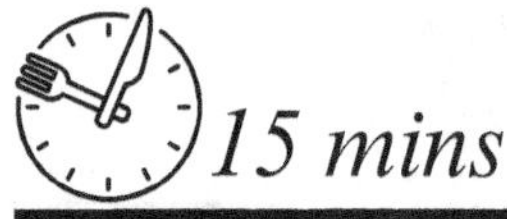 15 mins
 45 mins
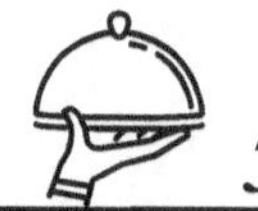 5

Prep time — *Cook time* — *Servings*

Ingredients

- 3 tablespoons extra virgin olive oil
- 1 medium yellow or white onion, chopped
- 3 carrots, peeled and chopped
- 2 celery stalks, chopped
- 1 to 2 cups chopped zucchini / yellow squash / bell pepper / sweet potatoes
- 6 garlic cloves minced
- ½ teaspoon dried thyme
- 1 large can (28 ounces) diced tomatoes
- 1 cup quinoa, rinsed well in a fine mesh colander (use less for a lighter, more broth-y soup)
- 4 cups (32 ounces) vegetable broth
- 2 cups water

Directions

1. In a large soup pot or Dutch oven, preheat the olive oil over medium heat. Add the chopped celery, carrot, onion, and other seasonal vegetables to the shimmering oil along with a dash of salt.
2. Cook for 6 to 8 minutes, stirring often, or until the onion is tender and starting to become translucent.
3. Add the thyme and garlic. Cook for approximately a minute, stirring often, or until aromatic. Add the chopped tomatoes along with their liquids and stir often for several more minutes.
4. Add the water, broth, and quinoa. Add two bay leaves, a sprinkle of red pepper flakes, and one teaspoon of salt. Add a lot of freshly ground black pepper for seasoning. Turn up the heat to a boil, cover the pot partially, and lower the heat to keep the mixture simmering gently.

- 1 teaspoon salt, more to taste
- 2 bay leaves
- Pinch red pepper flakes
- Freshly ground black pepper
- 1 can (15 ounces) great northern beans or chickpeas, rinsed and drained
- 1 cup or more chopped fresh kale or collard greens, tough ribs removed
- 1 to 2 teaspoons lemon juice, to taste
- Optional garnish: freshly grated Parmesan cheese

5. After cooking for 25 minutes, take off the top and mix in the chopped greens and beans. Simmer the greens for a further five minutes or until they are tender to your taste.

6. After turning off the heat, take out the bay leaves from the saucepan. Add one tsp of lemon juice and stir. Once the flavors are truly bursting, taste and adjust the seasoning with extra salt, pepper, and/or lemon juice.

7. You may require an additional ½ teaspoon of salt, based on your particular preferences and the type of vegetable broth you are using.

8. Transfer to a soup bowl and garnish with grated Parmesan cheese, if desired.

Nutrition facts per serving
Calories: 280 | Total Fat: 10.3g | Sodium 1019.4mg | Total Carbohydrate 40.8g | Dietary Fiber 8.9g | Sugars 9.2g | Protein 9g

Chicken and Rice Soup

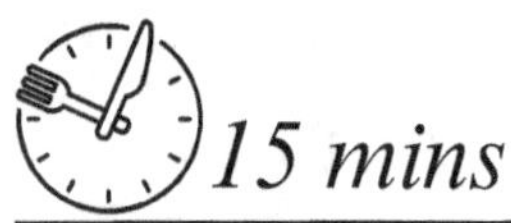 15 mins
Prep time

 45 mins
Cook time

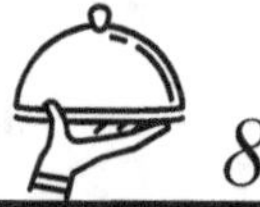 8
Servings

Ingredients

- 2 tbsp olive oil, or avocado oil
- 1 large onion, diced
- 2 large carrots, diced
- 1 stalk celery, diced
- 1 lb chicken breast (3 small), or chicken thighs
- 1/3 cup long grain rice, (uncooked) such as basmati or jasmine
- 8 cups chicken broth, or stock
- 1 cup water
- 1 tsp salt, adjust to taste
- 1/2 tsp ground black pepper, adjust to taste
- 2 bay leaves
- 2 tbsp fresh herbs, dill, or parsley, or a combination

Nutrition facts per serving
Calories: 174 | Fat: 7g | Sodium: 441mg | Carbohydrates: 12g | Fiber: 1g | Sugar: 2g | Protein: 18g

Directions

1. In a Dutch oven or soup pot set over medium heat, add the oil, then add the onion, carrots, and celery. Sauté for approximately 6-7 minutes, or until the vegetables are tender and starting to turn golden.
2. Add the rice, chicken, water, salt, pepper, and bay leaves to the chicken broth. Skim off any froth that comes to the top as you bring it to a boil.
3. Lower the heat to medium-low and gently boil the rice, covered, for 25 to 30 minutes, or until it becomes soft and the chicken is well cooked.
4. After taking the chicken out of the broth and shredding it into small pieces, return it to the soup and turn off the heat.
5. Add the herbs, taste, and adjust the seasoning, then serve.

80

Turkey & Barley Soup

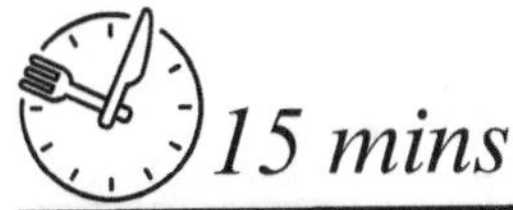 *15 mins*

 *25 mins*

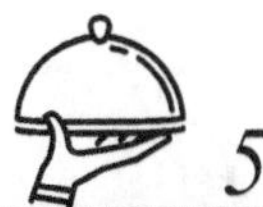 *5*

Prep time | *Cook time* | *Servings*

Ingredients

- 1 tbsp olive oil
- 1 medium onion, (peeled and diced)
- 2 medium carrots, diced (about 1 1/2 cups)
- 2 stalks celery (diced)
- 8 oz sliced mushrooms
- 1/2 cup of quick cooking barley
- 4 cups of fat-free low-sodium chicken broth
- 2 cups of water
- 2 cups (about 10 oz) cooked turkey breast (shredded or diced)
- 1/2 tsp salt
- 1/2 tsp ground black pepper

Nutrition facts per serving
Calories: 220 | Total Fat: 4.5g |
Sodium: 440mg | Total
Carbohydrate: 21g | Dietary:
Fiber 4g | Total Sugars: 5g |
Protein: 25g

Directions

1. In a soup pot set over medium-high heat, add the olive oil.
2. To the pot, add the mushrooms, celery, carrots, and onion. Add the onions and sauté for 8 to 10 minutes, or until they begin to turn translucent.
3. Stir in the water, broth, and barley. After bringing to a boil, lower the heat, and simmer for fifteen minutes.
4. Add little salt and pepper for seasoning. After the turkey is cooked through, serve.

Slow-Cooker Vegetable Minestrone Soup

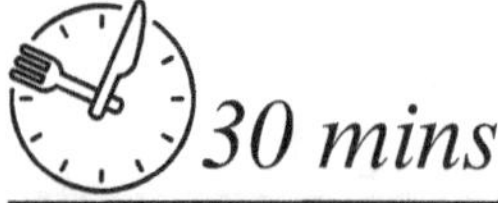 30 mins
Prep time

 6 hrs
Cook time

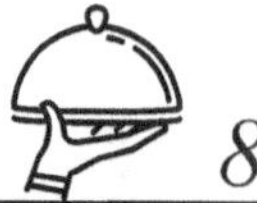 8
Servings

Ingredients

- 4 large carrots, peeled and chopped
- 3 stalks celery, chopped
- 1 small red onion, chopped
- 3 cloves garlic, minced
- 2 cups fresh green beans, trimmed and cut into 2-inch pieces
- 2 (15 ounce) cans no-sodium-added red kidney beans, rinsed
- 2 (15 ounce) cans no-sodium-added diced tomatoes, undrained
- 6 cups no-sodium-added vegetable broth
- 2 tablespoons Italian seasoning
- 1 teaspoon crushed red pepper
- ¾ teaspoon salt, divided
- ½ teaspoon ground pepper
- 1 large zucchini, chopped
- 4 ounces whole-wheat pasta elbows or other small pasta (about 1 cup)
- ½ cup freshly grated Parmesan cheese

Nutrition facts per serving
Calories: 222 | Total
Carbohydrate: 42g | Dietary
Fiber: 13g | Total Sugars: 10g |
Protein: 12g | Total Fat: 2g |
Sodium: 525mg

Directions

1. In a 6- to 8-quart slow cooker, combine the carrots, celery, onion, garlic, kidney beans, green beans, tomatoes, broth, Italian seasoning, crushed red pepper, 1/4 teaspoon salt, and pepper. Cook on low heat for 6 hours with a cover on.

2. Add the pasta, zucchini, and the last 1/2 teaspoon of salt. Cook the pasta on low for an additional 15 to 20 minutes, covered, or until it's soft.

3. Top each serving with approximately 1 1/2 teaspoons of Parmesan cheese and serve right away.

Spicy Chicken Noodle Soup with Soft-Boiled Eggs

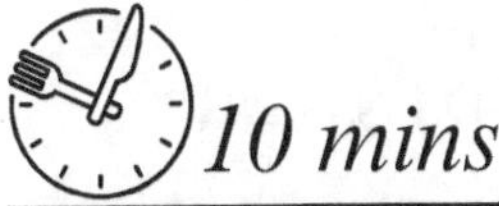 *10 mins*

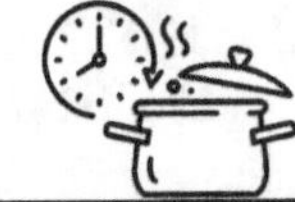

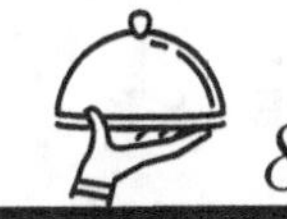 *8*

Prep time — *Cook time* — *Servings*

Ingredients

- 1 (10 ounce) can condensed low-sodium chicken noodle soup
- 1 ½ teaspoons grated fresh ginger
- ½ cup fresh cilantro leaves
- ½ cup grated carrot
- ¼ cup thinly sliced scallions
- 2 soft-boiled or hard-boiled eggs, halved
- 1/2 to 1 teaspoon Sriracha
- ½ teaspoon toasted sesame seeds

Directions

1. Make the soup as directed on the packet. Add the ginger and bring to a boil.
2. Split the soup between two shallow dishes that are broad. Add an egg, two tablespoons of scallions, and 1/4 cup of cilantro and carrot on top of each. Add some Sriracha and sesame seeds at the end.

Nutrition facts per serving
Calories: 175 | Total
Carbohydrate: 13g | Dietary
Fiber: 3g | Total Sugars: 5g |
Protein: 12g | Total Fat: 8g |
Sodium: 188mg

DAILY FOOD JOURNAL

DATE:

BREAKFAST	LUNCH	DESSERT	DINNER

TODAY'S WORKOUT

WATER INTAKE

NOTES

DAILY FOOD JOURNAL

DATE:

BREAKFAST	LUNCH	DESSERT	DINNER

TODAY'S WORKOUT

WATER INTAKE

NOTES

DAILY FOOD JOURNAL

DATE:

BREAKFAST	LUNCH	DESSERT	DINNER

TODAY'S WORKOUT

WATER INTAKE

NOTES

DAILY FOOD JOURNAL

DATE:

BREAKFAST	LUNCH	DESSERT	DINNER

TODAY'S WORKOUT

WATER INTAKE

NOTES

DAILY FOOD JOURNAL

DATE:

BREAKFAST	LUNCH	DESSERT	DINNER

TODAY'S WORKOUT

WATER INTAKE

NOTES

DAILY FOOD JOURNAL

DATE:

BREAKFAST	LUNCH	DESSERT	DINNER

TODAY'S WORKOUT

WATER INTAKE

NOTES

DAILY FOOD JOURNAL

DATE:

BREAKFAST	LUNCH	DESSERT	DINNER

TODAY'S WORKOUT

WATER INTAKE

NOTES

WEEKLY PLANNER

WEEK :

MONDAY

☐ ___________________________
☐ ___________________________
☐ ___________________________
☐ ___________________________

TUESDAY

☐ ___________________________
☐ ___________________________
☐ ___________________________
☐ ___________________________

WEDNESDAY

☐ ___________________________
☐ ___________________________
☐ ___________________________
☐ ___________________________

THURSDAY

☐ ___________________________
☐ ___________________________
☐ ___________________________
☐ ___________________________

FRIDAY

☐ ___________________________
☐ ___________________________
☐ ___________________________
☐ ___________________________

SATURDAY

☐ ___________________________
☐ ___________________________
☐ ___________________________
☐ ___________________________

SUNDAY

☐ ___________________________
☐ ___________________________
☐ ___________________________
☐ ___________________________

NOTE :

CHAPTER 8

LEGUMES AND PASTA

Coconut Flour Tortillas

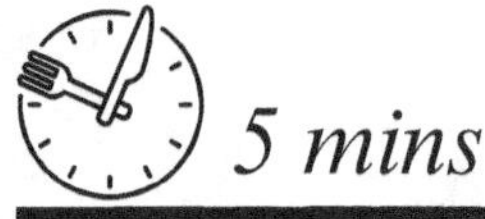 5 mins
Prep time

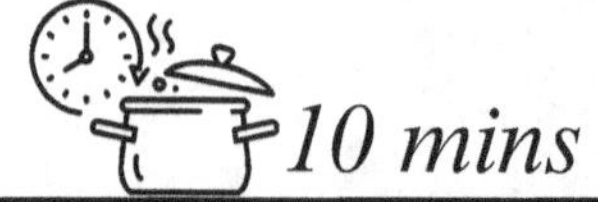 10 mins
Cook time

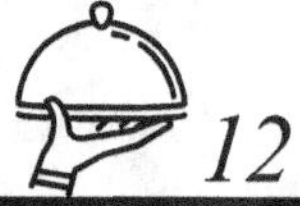 12
Servings

Ingredients

- 1/2 cup Coconut Flour
- 6 large Eggs
- 1 1/4 cups Almond milk or Coconut milk m
- 3/4 tsp Sea salt

Optional Add-in

- 1 tbsp Unflavored gelatin powder
- 1/2 tsp Cumin
- 1/2 tsp Paprika

Nutrition facts per serving
Calories: 64 | Fat: 3.5g |
Protein: 3.9g | Total Carbs: 3.8g
| Fiber: 1.9g | Sugar: 1.2g

Directions

1. Combine all ingredients in a large bowl and whisk until smooth. To allow for the natural thickening that comes from the coconut flour, let the batter sit for a minute or two. Just before frying, the batter should be extremely loose and flow readily; if necessary, add extra almond milk and eggs in equal quantities to achieve this.

2. Add the optional gelatin last if using it. Rather than pouring it all over the batter, sprinkle it on top and stir to prevent clumps. Next, pour in an additional 1/4 cup almond milk.

3. Grease a small pan (diameter of about 8 in.) gently with your preferred oil or with an oil mister and heat it over medium to medium-high heat. Transfer 1/4 cup (60 mL) of batter onto the skillet and tilt it quickly in various directions to distribute the batter evenly, just like you would while creating crepes.

4. Cook with a lid on until the edges become golden and little bubbles start to appear in the center. After you lift the lid, the edges will curl inward, taking one to two minutes. Turn, cover once again, and cook for a further one to two minutes, or until browned on the opposite side. Continue until all of the batter is utilized.

Pasta Puttanesca with Beef

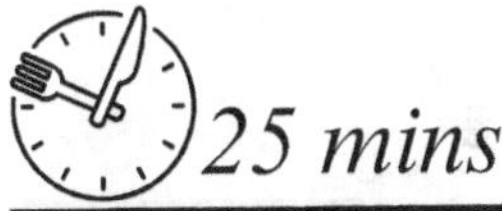 25 mins
Prep time

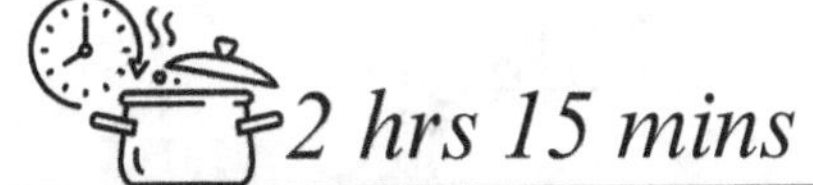 2 hrs 15 mins
Cook time

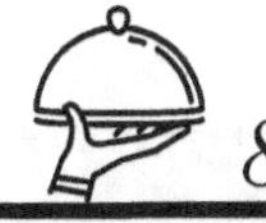 8
Servings

Ingredients

- 1 pound lean ground beef
- ¾ cup onion, chopped
- 4 cloves garlic, minced
- 2 (14.5 ounce) cans no-salt-added diced tomatoes, undrained
- 1 (6 ounce) can no-salt-added tomato paste
- 3 anchovy fillets, chopped
- 1 teaspoon dried oregano, crushed
- ¼ teaspoon crushed red pepper
- 8 ounces dried multigrain penne pasta (about 2 1/2 cups)
- ¼ cup Kalamata olives, chopped
- ¼ cup snipped fresh parsley
- 1 Snipped fresh parsley

Nutrition facts per serving
Calories: 262 | Total
Carbohydrate 31g | Dietary
Fiber: 5g | Total Sugars: 8g |
Protein: 19g | Total Fat: 8g |
Sodium: 215mg

Directions

1. Cook the ground beef, onion, and garlic in a large nonstick pan over medium heat until the meat is browned and the onion is soft. Remove fat and dispose of it.

2. Combine the meat mixture, tomatoes, tomato paste, anchovies, oregano, and crushed red pepper in a 4 or 3 1/2-quart slow cooker. Cook, covered, for four to six hours on low heat or two to three hours on high heat. As you wait, prepare the pasta as directed on the package and drain.

3. Stir in 1/4 cup parsley and olives before serving from the slow cooker. Over the hot, cooked pasta, serve the meat mixture. Garnish with more freshly chopped parsley, if preferred.

Chickpea Curry

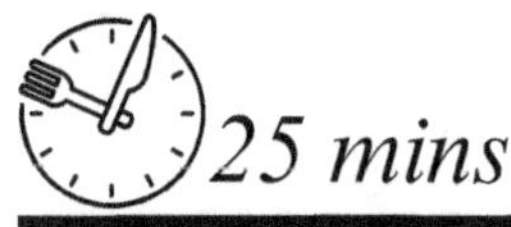 25 mins
Prep time

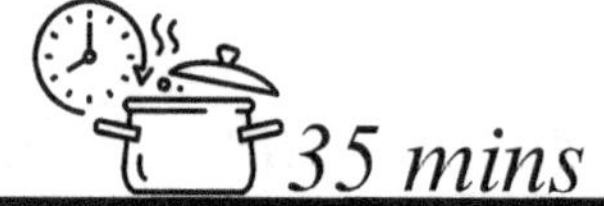 35 mins
Cook time

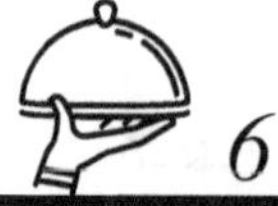 6
Servings

Ingredients

- 2 tablespoons avocado oil/olive oil
- 2 teaspoons coriander seeds
- 1 heaping teaspoon cumin seeds
- 15 to 20 fresh curry leaves
- 1 large yellow or red onion, finely diced
- 6 garlic cloves, minced
- 2- inch piece fresh ginger, minced or grated
- 1 to 3 serrano/jalapeno peppers, diced
- 2 tablespoons tomato paste
- ½ pound (227g) Roma or plum tomatoes (2 roma tomatoes), diced
- 2 teaspoons kosher salt
- 1 (13.5 oz /400 mL) can non-fat coconut milk
- ½ cup (120 mL) water
- 2 (15 oz /425g) cans chickpeas, drained and rinsed

Directions

1. For deglazing, keep a little basin of water close by.
2. In a medium-sized Dutch oven or 12-inch heavy-bottomed sauté pan, heat the oil over medium-high heat. When heated, add the coriander and cumin seeds and toss often for approximately a minute, or until fragrant and somewhat darker, being careful not to burn them!
3. Add the curry leaves and cover the pan right away, take a step back to avoid spilling oil. Just cook for 20 seconds to avoid scorching.
4. Add the onions and a pinch teaspoon of salt. Cook for 5 minutes, or until the onions begin to change color. Reduce the heat to medium if the spices begin to darken. If necessary, add a dash of water to keep the onions from browning.
5. Add the ginger, garlic, and serrano/jalapeno peppers. Cook, stirring constantly, for one to two minutes.

- 3 tablespoons tahini, well-stirred
- 1/2 teaspoon brown sugar, or coconut sugar
- 1 small head of Swiss chard or lacinato kale
- 2 teaspoons garam masala
- Freshly squeezed lemon or lime juice, ½ to 1 tablespoon, to taste
- 1 big handful of cilantro leaves and tender stems, chopped
- 1 big handful of fresh mint leaves, chopped

Ground spices
- 1 ½ teaspoons curry powder
- 1 teaspoon ground coriander
- ½ teaspoon ground cinnamon
- 1/2 teaspoon freshly grated nutmeg
- ¼ teaspoon ground turmeric
- A generous amount of freshly cracked black pepper

Nutrition facts per serving
Calories: 360 | Carbohydrates: 33g | Protein: 12g | Fat: 22g | Sodium: 1352mg | Fiber: 10g | Sugar: 4g

6. For 90 seconds, mix constantly after adding the tomato paste and ground spices. Sprinkle in some water if it starts to dry out.

7. Add two teaspoons of kosher salt and the tomatoes. To remove burned parts, scrape up tomato juice. Simmer the tomatoes for 5 minutes, or until they are tender and the oil begins to come out of them.

8. Add the sugar, tahini, coconut milk, water, and chickpeas. Give it a good stir and simmer. For fifteen to twenty minutes, simmer with a lid on, periodically opening the pot to stir.

9. Rinse the mint, cilantro, and Swiss chard (or kale) in the meantime. Remove and discard the middle ribs from the greens. Roll up the leaves, then finely slice them. Chop the mint and cilantro.

10. Add the greens after the simmering period. Simmer for 4 to 5 minutes, or until tender and wilted. Add the garam masala and stir to mix.

11. Squeeze in some lime or lemon juice, cilantro, and mint after turning off the heat. Add salt (approximately ½ teaspoon kosher salt) to taste. Let the flavors merge by resting for five to fifteen minutes. Accompany with warm rice or pita bread.

Cauliflower Rice

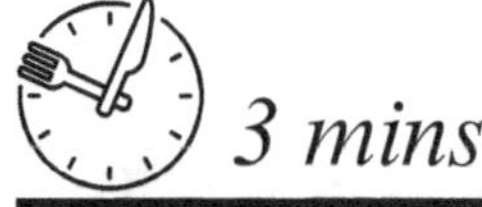 *3 mins*
Prep time

 *7 mins*
Cook time

 4
Servings

Ingredients

- 1 fresh medium cauliflower
- Good handful coriander, chopped
- Cumin seeds, toasted (optional)

Directions

1. Remove the tough center and stems from the cauliflower, then pulse the remaining parts in a food processor until the grains resemble rice.
2. Transfer into a heatproof dish, place cling film over it, puncture it, and cook in the microwave for 7 minutes on high without adding any water.
3. Incorporate the coriander. Toast some cumin seeds to give some spice to the rice.

Nutrition facts per serving
Calories: 25 | Total Fat: 0.3g |
Sodium: 30mg | Total
Carbohydrates: 5g | Dietary
Fiber: 2g | Sugars: 3g | Protein:
3g

Mediterranean Chickpea Salad

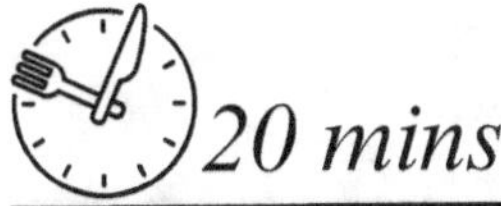 *20 mins*
Prep time

Cook time

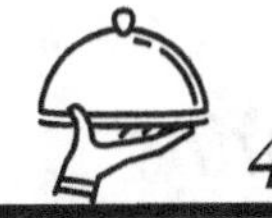 *4*
Servings

Ingredients

- 2 tablespoons extra-virgin olive oil
- 3 garlic cloves, minced
- 1 tablespoon lemon zest
- 2 tablespoons lemon juice
- 3/4 teaspoon sea salt
- Freshly ground black pepper
- 1 ½ teaspoon cumin seeds
- 2 cups cooked chickpeas, drained and rinsed
- 1 cup cherry tomatoes, halved
- 4 Medjool dates, pitted and diced
- 3 Persian cucumbers, sliced into thin half moons
- ⅓ cup chopped roasted red peppers
- ¼ cup finely chopped parsley
- 3 ounces Roth Chèvre Honey Goat Cheese
- ¼ cup fresh mint
- ⅓ cup roasted chickpeas, optional

Directions

1. Combine the olive oil, garlic, lemon zest, lemon juice, salt, and pepper to taste in a large mixing basin.

2. Toast the cumin seeds in a small pan over medium-low heat for 30 seconds, or until fragrant. Remove them from the fire and lightly smash them (a mortar and pestle works best for this). Add them to the bowl and mix well.

3. Toss in the chickpeas, tomatoes, dates, cucumbers, red pepper, and parsley. Transfer to a serving tray and top with the goat cheese, mint, and more roasted chickpeas, if preferred. Season with salt and pepper to taste, then serve.

Nutrition facts per serving
Calories: 498 | Fat: 28g | Carbohydrates: 43.7g | Fiber: 9.6g | Sugar: 4g | Protein: 15.8 grams | Sodium: 567mg

Tortilla Chip Flounder with Black Bean Salad

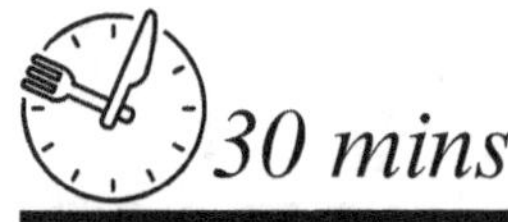 30 mins
 10 mins
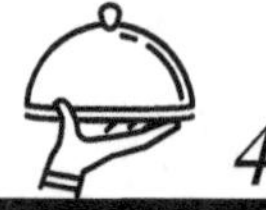 4

Prep time   *Cook time*   *Servings*

Ingredients

- 4 (3-4) ounce fresh or frozen flounder fillets or other white fish fillets
- Cooking spray
- 4 ounces multi-grain tortilla chips
- 1/8-1/4 teaspoon cayenne pepper
- ⅓ cup refrigerated or frozen egg product, thawed
- 1 (15 ounce) can no-salt-added black beans, rinsed and drained
- ½ cup halved cherry tomatoes
- ½ cup chopped green bell pepper
- ¼ cup finely chopped red onion
- 2 tablespoons chopped fresh oregano

Directions

1. If the fish is frozen, thaw it first. Preheat the oven to 425°F. Using foil, line a baking pan. Spray cooking spray on the foil and lay aside the baking sheet.

2. In a food processor, combine the tortilla chips and the cayenne pepper. Process, covered, until very finely crushed. Pour into a shallow dish.

3. Rinse and pat dry the fish. Pour the egg into a separate shallow dish. Dip the fish in the egg, then in the crumbled tortilla chips, coat it. Place the fish on the baking sheet that has been preheated. Spray the top of the fish lightly with cooking spray. Bake for 8–10 minutes, or until the fish flakes easily with a fork.

- 2 tablespoons chopped fresh Italian parsley plus more for garnish
- 1 tablespoon lemon juice
- 2 teaspoons olive oil
- ¼ teaspoon salt
- ¼ teaspoon ground cumin
- ¼ cup crumbled queso fresco (1 ounce)
- 1 sprig Chopped fresh Italian parsley

4. In the meantime, in a medium mixing bowl, add black beans, tomatoes, bell pepper, onion, oregano, 2 tablespoons parsley, lemon juice, oil, salt, and cumin. Place the fish on top of the bean salad and serve. Sprinkle with cheese and parsley, if preferred.

Nutrition facts per serving
Serving Size 1 fillet and 2/3 cup bean salad
Calories: 361 | Total Carbohydrate: 36g
Dietary Fiber: 8g | Total Sugars: 3g |
Protein: 28g | Total Fat: 11g | Sodium: 401mg

Spaghetti with Tomato and Basil

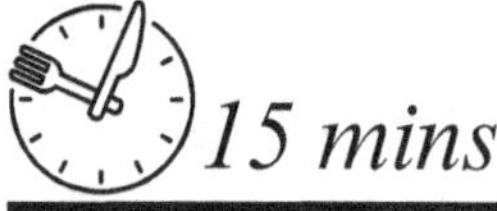 15 mins
Prep time

 25 mins
Cook time

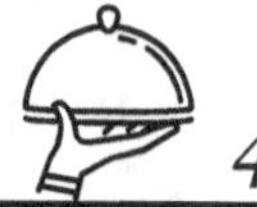 4
Servings

Ingredients

- 3 pounds fresh plum tomatoes, blanched, peeled seeded and quartered
- 3 ounces olive oil
- Salt and freshly ground pepper to taste
- 1 pinch crushed red-pepper flakes
- 1 pound dry spaghetti
- 2 ounces extra-virgin olive oil
- 1 tablespoon butter
- 6 leaves fresh basil, shredded
- 2 tablespoons freshly grated Parmigiano-Reggiano cheese

Nutrition facts per serving
Calories: 350 | Total Fat: 16g |
Sodium: 250mg | Total
Carbohydrates: 45g | Dietary
Fiber: 4g | Sugars: 6g | Protein:
10g

Directions

1. Blanch the tomatoes and peel off the skins. Cut it in half lengthwise and scrape out the seeds. The tomatoes should be cut crosswise. Place in a dish and set aside.

2. In a large, deep pan over medium-high heat, heat 3 ounces of olive oil until it smokes slightly. Add the tomatoes, salt, pepper, and crushed red pepper. Because the tomatoes will diminish and the salt will become more concentrated, season with a gentler touch at first.

3. With a potato masher, crush the tomatoes until they are in fine bits and all of their juice has been released. To make a semi-chunky sauce, make sure they're finely chopped and smashed. Simmer for 25 minutes over medium heat.

4. As the sauce simmers, cook the pasta in salted water until it's halfway done. Drain while retaining some of the water.

5. Taste the sauce and adjust the spices as needed. Cook the pasta in the sauce over medium-high heat until all of the liquid is absorbed and the pasta is al dente. If the sauce is too thick, add more pasta liquid to thin it up.

6. Remove the skillet from the heat and add the extra-virgin olive oil, butter, basil, and cheese. Mix until the spaghetti has an orangey hue. Taste again and adjust the salt if required. Transfer to a plate. Serve.

Black Bean Tacos

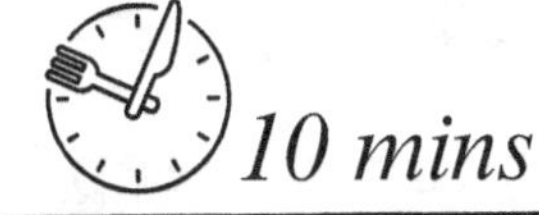 *10 mins*

 *15 mins*

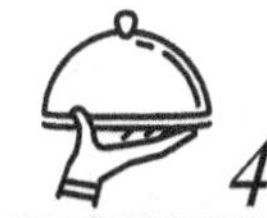 *4*

Prep time | *Cook time* | *Servings*

Ingredients

- 2 (15 ounce) cans black beans, rinsed
- 1 teaspoon ground cumin
- ½ teaspoon garlic powder
- 8 hard taco shells
- ¾ cup shredded Mexican cheese blend

Nutrition facts per serving
Serving Size 2 tacos
Calories: 328 | Total
Carbohydrate: 42g | Dietary
Fiber: 10g | Total Sugars: 6g |
Protein: 15g | Total Fat: 11g |
Sodium: 299mg

Directions

1. Preheat the oven to 325 degrees Fahrenheit.
2. In a large mixing basin, mash half of the beans. Stir in the entire beans, cumin, and garlic powder. Fill each taco shell halfway with the bean mixture. Serve with cheese on top.
3. Place the filled tacos on a baking sheet and bake for 12 to 15 minutes, or until the beans are heated and the cheese is melted.

Shrimp Scampi

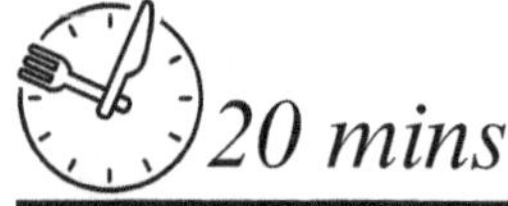 *20 mins*

Prep time

Cook time

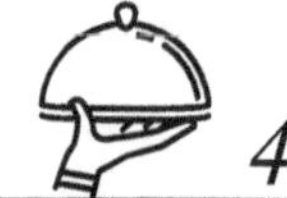 *4*

Servings

Ingredients

- 1 ½ pounds fresh or frozen large shrimp in shells
- 6 ounces whole-wheat or plain linguine
- 1 tablespoon olive oil
- 3 cloves garlic, minced
- 2 tablespoons dry white wine or reduced-sodium chicken broth
- 1 tablespoon butter
- ⅛ teaspoon salt
- 1 tablespoon chopped fresh chives or parsley

Nutrition facts per serving
Calories: 341 | Total
Carbohydrate: 34g | Dietary
Fiber: 1g | Total Sugars: 2g |
Protein: 29g | Total Fat: 9g |
Sodium: 250mg

Directions

1. If using frozen shrimp, thaw them first. If desired, leave shrimp tails intact after peeling and deveining. Rinse shrimp and wipe dry with paper towels.
2. Cook the linguine according to the package guidelines. Drain and keep warm.
3. Meanwhile, place a 12-inch skillet over medium-high heat with oil. Cook and stir for 15 seconds after adding garlic. Serve with shrimp. Cook for 2 to 4 minutes, or until shrimp become opaque, stirring often. With a slotted spoon, transfer the shrimp to a serving plate.
4. In the skillet, combine the wine (or reduced-sodium chicken broth), butter, and salt. Cook and stir over medium heat to release any browned parts and melt the butter. Pour the butter mixture over the shrimp. Sprinkle with chives. Serve with linguine.

104

Brown Rice and Vegetable Stir-fry

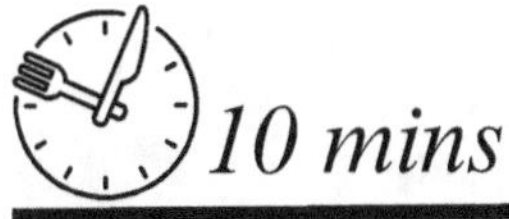 *10 mins*
Prep time

 *35 mins*
Cook time

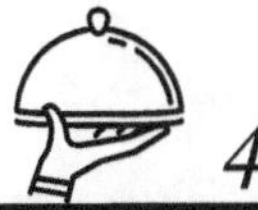 *4*
Servings

Ingredients

- ½ cup uncooked brown rice
- 1 cup red cabbage, chopped
- ½ head of broccoli, chopped
- ½ red bell pepper, chopped
- ½ zucchini, chopped
- 2 tablespoon extra virgin olive oil
- 4 cloves of garlic, minced
- 1 handful fresh parsley, finely chopped
- ⅛ teaspoon cayenne powder
- 2 tablespoon tamari or soy sauce
- Sesame seeds for garnish, optional

Nutrition facts per serving
Calories: 197 | Carbohydrates: 28.1g | Protein: 5.6g | Fat: 7.9g | Sodium: 476.8mg | Fiber: 4.1g | Sugar: 3.5g

Directions

1. Brown rice should be cooked according to package recommendations.
2. In a wok or frying pan, bring some water to a boil. Then, over high heat, add the vegetables (they must be covered by water) and cook for 1 to 2 minutes. Drain and put aside the vegetables.
3. In a wok, heat the oil and add the garlic, cayenne pepper, and parsley. Cook for about 1 minute over high heat, stirring periodically.
4. Add in the veggies, rice, and tamari, cook for another 1 to 2 minutes.
5. Garnish with sesame seeds (optional).
6. Refrigerate the brown rice stir-fry in an airtight container for up to 5 days.

105

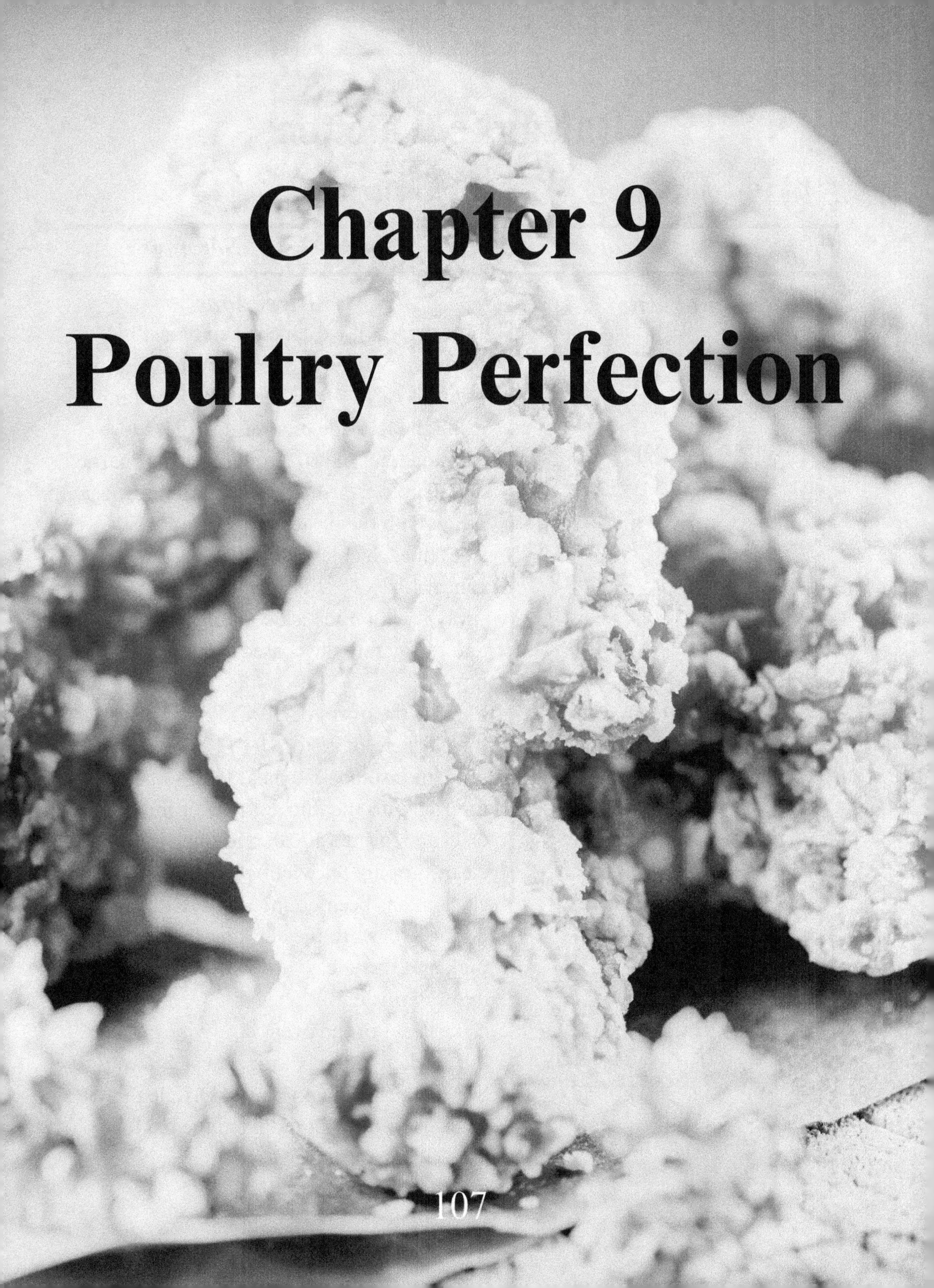

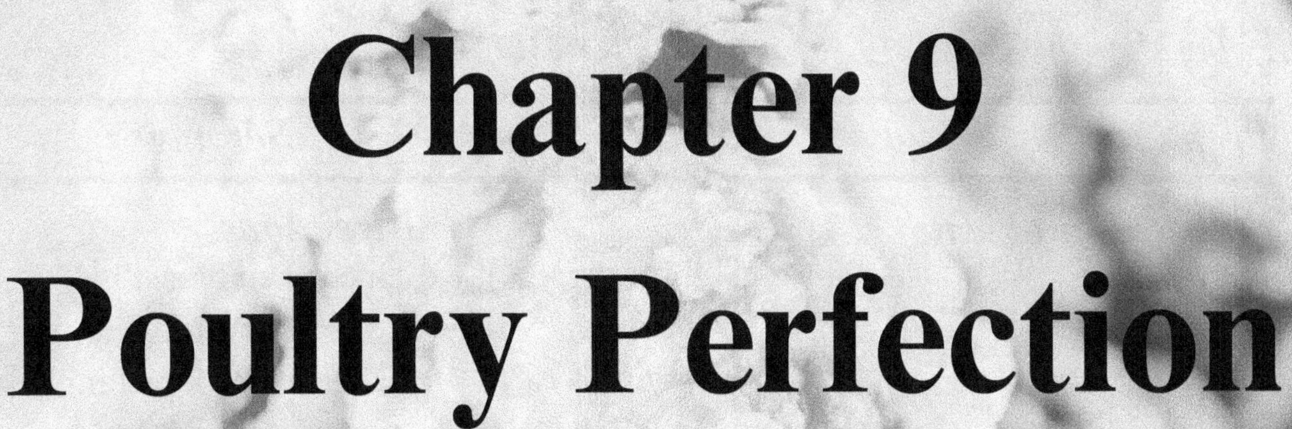

Chapter 9
Poultry Perfection

Balsamic Chicken

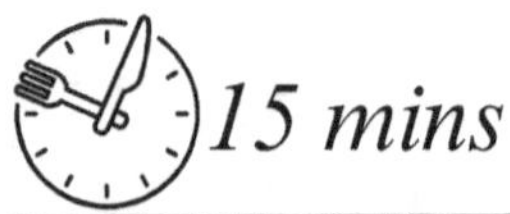 15 mins

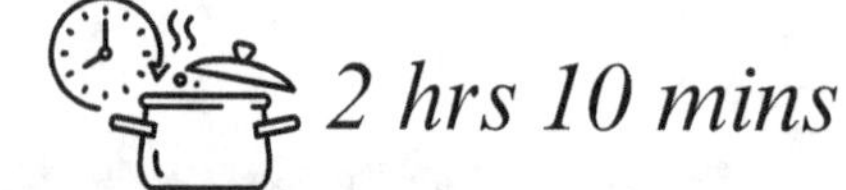 2 hrs 10 mins

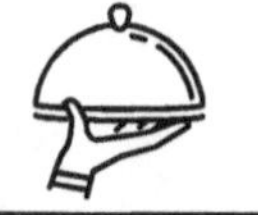 4

| Prep time | Cook time | Servings |

Ingredients

- 4 (4 ounce) skinless, boneless chicken breast halves
- 1 tablespoon paprika
- 1 tablespoon olive oil
- ½ teaspoon snipped fresh rosemary
- 2 cloves garlic, minced
- ¼ teaspoon ground black pepper
- Nonstick cooking spray
- ¼ cup dry red wine or water
- 3 tablespoons balsamic vinegar
- 4 sprigs Fresh rosemary sprigs

Nutrition facts per serving
Calories: 181 | Total
Carbohydrate: 3g | Dietary
Fiber: 1g | Total Sugars: 0g |
Protein: 27g | Total Fat: 5g |
Sodium: 62mg

Directions

1. If preferred, lay each chicken breast half between two pieces of plastic wrap and pound to a 1/4- to 1/2-inch-thick rectangle using the flat side of a meat mallet.
2. Mix together paprika, oil, rosemary, garlic, and pepper in a small bowl until it forms a paste. Rub the paste mixture onto both sides of each chicken breast.
3. Line a 13x9x2-inch baking dish with foil or spray it with nonstick cooking spray. Cover and refrigerate the coated chicken for 2 to 6 hours.
4. Preheat the oven to 450°F. Pour wine over the chicken. Bake for 10 to 12 minutes, or until an instant-read meat thermometer inserted into the thickest part of the chicken registers 170°F and the juices flow clear, flipping once halfway through. (If the chicken has been pounded, bake for 6 minutes, or until the chicken is no longer pink and the juices run clear, flipping midway through.)
5. Take it out of the oven. Pour vinegar over the chicken in the baking pan right away. Serve the chicken on plates. Drizzle the chicken with the liquid from the baking pan. Garnish with fresh rosemary, if using.

Chicken and Broccoli Stir-fry

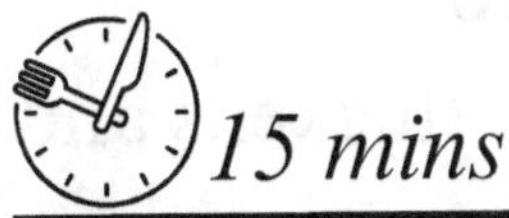 15 mins
 15 mins
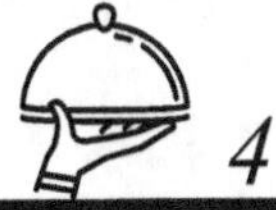 4

Prep time · Cook time · Servings

Ingredients

Chicken and Broccoli:
- 1 lb chicken breast, (boneless skinless), cut into 3/4" pieces
- 2 Tbsp cooking oil, (I used extra light olive oil), divided
- 1 lb broccoli, cut into florets (about 5 cups)
- 1 small yellow onion, sliced into strips
- 1/2 lb white button mushrooms, thickly sliced

Stir Fry Sauce Ingredients:
- 2/3 cup low sodium chicken broth
- 3 Tbsp low sodium soy sauce, (use Tamari for gluten free), or added to taste
- 2 Tbsp light brown sugar, packed (or honey to taste)
- 1 Tbsp cornstarch
- 1 Tbsp sesame oil

Directions

1. Combine all of the sauce ingredients in a small dish and whisk to dissolve the sugar and cornstarch (warm broth will help the sugar dissolve faster). Set aside the sauce.

2. Chicken should be cut into small bite-sized pieces (no more than 3/4" thick) and gently seasoned with pepper. Medium-high heat in a large, heavy skillet or wok. Add 1 tablespoon of oil. Allow the chicken to remain in a single layer for 1 minute to sear, then stir fry for another 5 minutes, or until golden brown and cooked through. Transfer to a bowl and loosely cover to keep warm.

3. Add 1 tablespoon of oil to the same skillet, along with the broccoli florets, sliced onion, and sliced mushrooms. Reduce heat to medium/low after 3 minutes, or until mushrooms have softened and broccoli is crisp-tender.

- 1 tsp fresh ginger, peeled and grated (lightly packed)
- 1 tsp garlic (2 small cloves), grated
- 1/4 tsp black pepper, plus more to season chicken

4. Give the sauce a brief toss to ensure there is no starch, and then pour it all over the veggies. Simmer for 3–4 minutes, or until the sauce thickens and the flavors of the garlic and ginger have mellowed. Add water a spoonful at a time to thin the sauce.

5. Return the chicken to the pan and cook for another 30 seconds, or until well heated. Serve over hot rice with additional soy sauce to taste.

Nutrition facts per serving
Calories: 325 | Fat: 14g |
Sodium: 586mg |
Carbohydrates: 21g | Fiber: 4g |
Sugar: 10g | Protein: 31g

Chicken Casserole

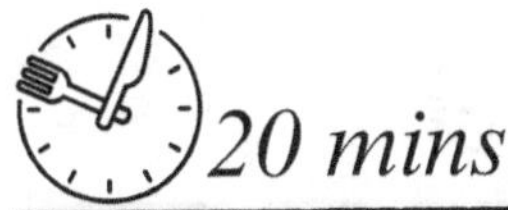 *20 mins*
Prep time

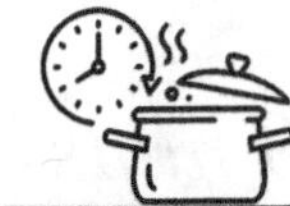 *50 mins*
Cook time

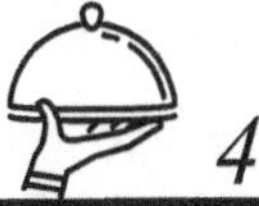 *4*
Servings

Ingredients

- 4 small skinless chicken breasts (500g)
- 1 large onion, chopped
- 2 garlic cloves, crushed
- 2 green peppers, seeded and chopped
- 2 tbsp fresh marjoram or half tbsp dried
- 400g (1) tin chopped tomatoes
- 150ml low-salt chicken stock
- 420g (1) can borlotti beans, drained and rinsed
- 2 tbsp tomato purée
- Freshly ground black pepper

Nutrition facts per serving
Calories: 274 | Carbs: 16.3g |
Fiber: 16.0g | Protein: 38.6g |
Fat: 2.5g | Sugars: 10.2g

Directions

1. Sauté the chicken breasts until brown on both sides in a large nonstick skillet. If the chicken is sticking to the pan, add a little water.
2. Continue to sauté for 2-3 minutes after adding the onion, garlic, and peppers.
3. Mix in the diced tomatoes, chicken stock, beans, tomato puree, freshly ground pepper, and herbs.
4. Stir thoroughly, bring to a boil, cover, and leave to cook for 40–45 minutes.

Turkey meatballs with zucchini noodles

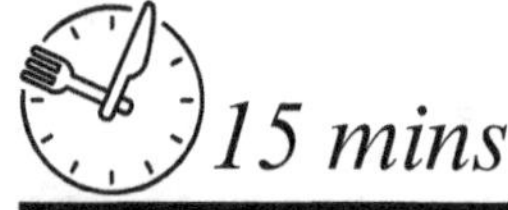 *15 mins*
 *20 mins*
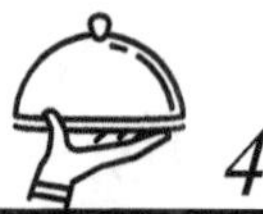 *4*

Prep time — **Cook time** — **Servings**

Ingredients

Meatballs
- Nonstick spray
- 1 tablespoon extra-virgin olive oil
- 1 sweet onion, minced
- 2 garlic cloves, minced
- ¼ cup fresh chopped parsley
- 3 tablespoons grated Parmesan cheese
- 1 pound ground turkey
- ¾ teaspoon kosher salt
- ½ teaspoon freshly ground black pepper

Sides
- 3 pounds zucchini, spiralized
- ½ teaspoon kosher salt
- 2 cups marinara sauce
- Parmesan cheese, as needed for garnishing

Directions

1. Set the oven to 375°F in order to prepare the meatballs. Apply nonstick spray after lining a baking pan with aluminum foil.

2. Heat the olive oil in a medium-sized pan over medium heat. Add the onion and cook for approximately 5 minutes, or until soft. Add the garlic and cook for a further minute or until fragrant.

3. Pour the mixture into a medium bowl and let it cool down a bit. Add the turkey, parsley, and Parmesan cheeses and stir. Season with salt and pepper. Roll the ingredients into ball shapes (approximately 2 tablespoons per ball) and place them on the baking sheet that has been prepared.

4. After putting the baking sheet in the oven, bake the meatballs for 17 to 20 minutes, or until they are done.

5. Make the Zucchini Noodles: Place the zucchini in a large colander, mix with salt, and let rest for five minutes while the meatballs cook.

6. Heat a big saucepan of salted water until it boils. After soaking the zucchini for a minute, strain it well.

7. Divide the zucchini noodles into four containers (or plates) for assembly or serving. Place meatballs and ½ cup of marinara sauce on top. Add Parmesan as a garnish.

8. Serve right away or store in the fridge for up to four days.

Nutrition facts per serving
Calories: 393 | Fat: 18g | Carbs: 28g | Protein: 33g | Sugars: 20g

Oven Roasted Turkey reast

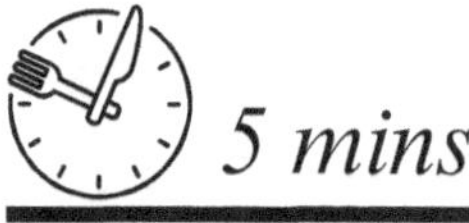 **5 mins**

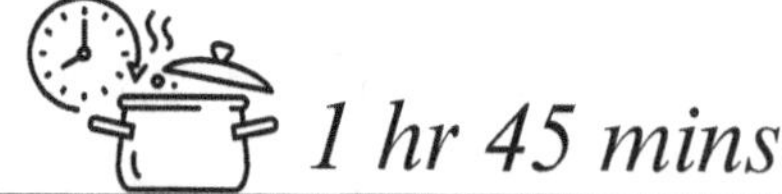 **1 hr 45 mins**

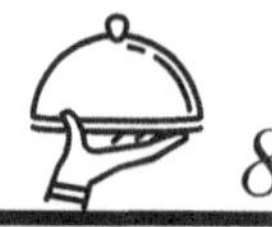 **8**

Prep time   *Cook time*   *Servings*

Ingredients

- 2 tablespoons olive oil
- 2 teaspoons paprika
- 2 teaspoons dried oregano
- 2 teaspoons dried rosemary minced
- 2 teaspoons salt
- 1 teaspoon dried thyme
- 1 teaspoon black pepper
- 1 teaspoon onion powder
- 1 teaspoon garlic powder
- 3 to 8 pound turkey breast

Nutrition facts per serving
Calories: 151 | Carbohydrates:
1g | Protein: 25g | Fat: 5g |
Sodium: 816mg | Fiber: 1g |
Sugar: 1g

Directions

1. Preheat the oven to 375°F. Place the turkey breast, skin side up, on a roasting pan rack or in a lightly oiled 9x13 pan.
2. In a small bowl, whisk together the olive oil, paprika, oregano, rosemary, salt, thyme, black pepper, onion powder, and garlic powder to produce a paste.
3. With your finger, loosen the skin and put some of the spice mixture below it. Smooth it over the meat to cover as much as possible. Rub the leftover spice mixture over the skin of the turkey breast.
4. Cook for about 20 minutes per pound in a preheated oven, or until the turkey reaches an internal temperature of 160 degrees Fahrenheit. The temperature should be taken in the middle of the thickest region of the breast.
5. The cooking time will vary depending on the size of your turkey breast. Boneless turkey breasts will cook more quickly. To ensure accuracy, use a meat thermometer.
6. Remove from the oven and cover with aluminum foil to keep warm. Allow for a 15-minute rest until the internal temperature reaches 165°F. Then cut and serve.

Garlic Chicken thighs

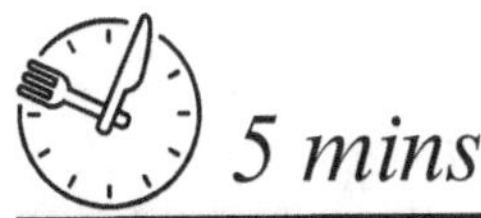 **5 mins**

Prep time

 **15 mins**

Cook time

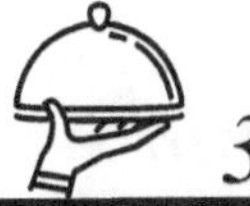 **3**

Servings

Ingredients

- 6 Boneless skinless chicken thighs
- ½ tablespoon paprika
- ½ teaspoon ground black pepper
- 2 tablespoons unsalted butter
- 2 tablespoons olive oil
- 5 garlic cloves crushed
- ⅓ cup low sodium chicken stock substitute with white wine
- 1 teaspoon salt or use according to preference

Nutrition facts per serving
Calories: 430 | Carbohydrates: 3g | Protein: 44g | Fat: 26g | Sodium: 979mg | Fiber: 1g | Sugar: 1g

Directions

1. Using a kitchen towel, pat dry the chicken thighs, then cut off any extra or noticeable fat and set them aside. To ensure consistent cooking, let the chicken thighs come to room temperature before cooking.
2. In a small bowl, add paprika, salt, and black pepper. Mix the chicken thighs with the dry rub (chicken marinade) until well combined.
3. Heat a pan over medium heat, add the butter and olive oil, and cook until the butter melts. Add the smashed garlic and cook for approximately 2 minutes, or until it softens and releases aroma.
4. Sear the chicken thighs for approximately 4 minutes on each side after adding them to the heated garlic oil. If necessary, deglaze the pan by moving around after adding the chicken stock.
5. To ensure that the pan sauce coats both sides, flip the chicken thighs once. Cook for a further two minutes, or until the internal temperature reaches 165F/73C and it's well cooked.
6. Remove from the fire, add some chopped parsley and lemon slices, and serve right away.

115

Grounded Beef with Vegetable Stir-fry

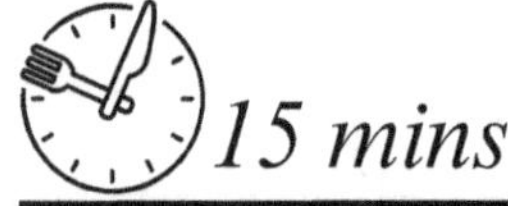 *15 mins*
Prep time

 *15 mins*
Cook time

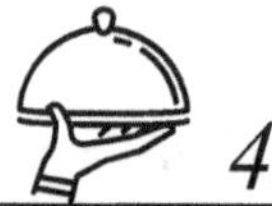 *4*
Servings

Ingredients

Meat seasoning

- Heap ¼ teaspoon each: garlic salt, onion powder, celery salt, black pepper

Sauce

- 3 Tablespoons cornstarch, + 3 tbsp. cold water
- 1 cup beef broth
- ½ cup chicken broth
- ¼ cup soy sauce
- ¼ cup honey, can sub brown sugar
- 3 cloves garlic, minced
- 1 teaspoon hot sauce
- ¼ tsp ground ginger

Stir-fry

- 1 ¼ lbs. ground beef
- 2 tablespoons peanut oil, can sub olive or vegetable oil
- 1/3 cup dry white wine, or beef broth.
- 2 cups broccoli florets
- 1 cup green beans

Directions

1. In a closed container, add cornstarch and cold water and shake to blend. Set it away in a cool place.
2. Set aside the remaining sauce ingredients in a medium bowl.
3. Before you begin, measure out the remaining ingredients.
4. Season the beef. In a large pan, heat the olive oil over medium-high heat. Cook and shred the ground meat until browned and cooked thoroughly. Set aside.
5. Set the heat to medium and add the white wine. Use a silicone spatula to "clean" the bottom and sides of the skillet. Cook until the liquid has been reduced by half, about 3 minutes.
6. If necessary, add a dash of more oil. Toss in the broccoli, green beans, mushrooms, onions, and celery.

116

- 8 oz. mushrooms
- 1 small yellow onion, sliced
- ½ cup carrots, julienned
- ½ red bell pepper, sliced
- 1 rib celery, diced
- For Serving
- 3 cups of cooked rice, any kind(for serving).

Cook for 3 minutes, or until slightly softened. Cook for 2 minutes with the carrots and bell peppers.

7. Bring the sauce mixture to a low boil. Allow it to simmer or reduce for 2-3 minutes. Shake the cornstarch mixture vigorously. Slowly whisk the cornstarch slurry into the simmering sauce until the appropriate thickness is achieved. Reduce the heat to low.

8. Return the ground beef to the skillet, along with any juices from the dish. Allow it to cook through in the sauce, approximately 2 minutes. Garnish with your favorite toppings and serve with rice or noodles.

Nutrition facts per serving
Calories: 437 | Carbohydrates: 37g | Protein: 37g | Fat: 15g | Sodium: 1353mg | Fiber: 4g | Sugar: 23g

Grilled Lemon Herb Chicken

 *1 hr*
Prep time

 *15 mins*
Cook time

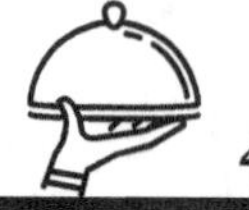 *4*
Servings

Ingredients

- 2 lbs chicken breasts, trimmed
- 1/4 cup olive oil, extra virgin
- 1/4 cup lemon juice
- 1 tbsp dried basil
- 1 tbsp dried parsley
- 1 tsp salt
- 1/2 tsp black pepper
- 1/2 tsp garlic powder
- 1/2 tsp onion powder
- 1/4 tsp crushed red pepper flakes

Nutrition facts per serving
Calories: 388 | Carbohydrates: 2g | Protein: 49g | Fat: 20g | Sodium: 850mg | Fiber: 1g | Sugar: 1g

Directions

1. In a small mixing bowl, combine the oil, black pepper, garlic powder, red pepper flakes, onion powder, parsley, basil, and salt.
2. Place the chicken breasts in a gallon Ziploc bag with the lemon herb marinade ingredients. Squeeze out any extra air when you seal the bag. Marinade the chicken for at least one hour and up to 12 hours.
3. Depending on your preference, you can grill or sauté your chicken. I've included directions for each of them below.
4. TO BE GRILLED: Remove each chicken breast from the bag and lay it on a hot, medium-heated grill. 5–7 minutes per side, or until done.

5. IN THE STOVE: In a skillet over medium heat, add 2 tablespoons of olive oil or another cooking fat. Heat the oil over medium-high heat. (When the chicken sizzles when you place it in the pan, it's done.) Arrange the chicken breasts in a single layer in the skillet. 5 minutes. You should flip your chicken. Cook for 5 minutes more. (When finished, the chicken should be firm to the touch, and the juices should run clear).

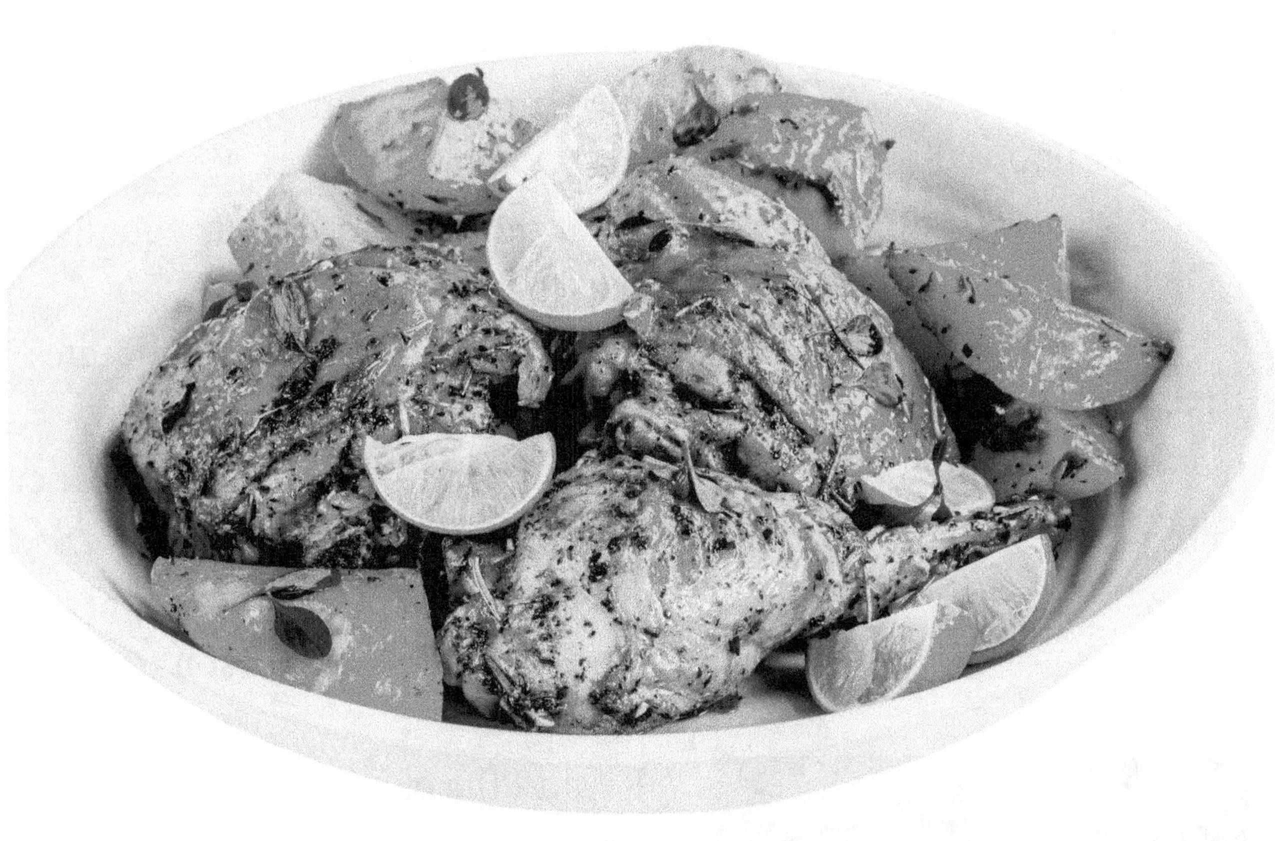

Lemon Pepper Chicken

 *8 mins*

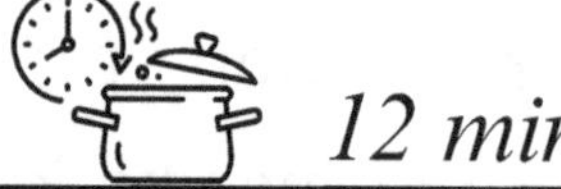 *12 mins*

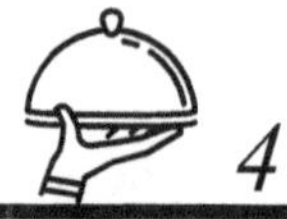 *4*

| *Prep time* | *Cook time* | *Servings* |

Ingredients

- 4 thin cut boneless skinless chicken breasts
- 1/3 cup all purpose flour
- 1 tablespoon lemon pepper seasoning or more to taste
- salt to taste
- 2 tablespoons olive oil
- 2 tablespoons butter
- 2 teaspoons lemon juice
- 1 tablespoon chopped parsley
- sliced lemons and parsley sprigs optional garnish

Nutrition facts per serving
Calories: 345 | Carbohydrates: 11g | Protein: 36g | Fat: 17g | Sodium: 1000mg | Fiber: 1g | Sugar: 1g

Directions

1. Combine the flour, lemon pepper spice, and salt and pepper to taste. Fill a small basin or plate with the flour mixture.
2. In a large saucepan set over medium-high heat, heat the olive oil.
3. Coat the chicken breasts equally in the flour mixture.
4. Cook the chicken for 5–6 minutes per side or until done.
5. Place the chicken on a dish and set it aside. To remain warm, cover
6. In the pan, melt the butter and mix in the lemon juice. Season to taste with salt.
7. Re-add the chicken to the pan. Pour the sauce over the chicken.
8. Garnish with lemon slices and additional parsley sprigs, if preferred, and serve.

Baked Chicken with Onions & Leeks

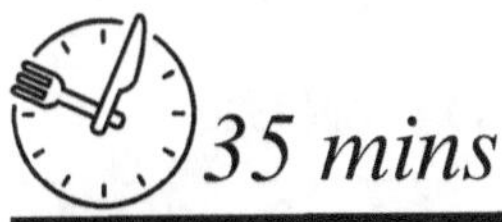 35 mins
Prep time

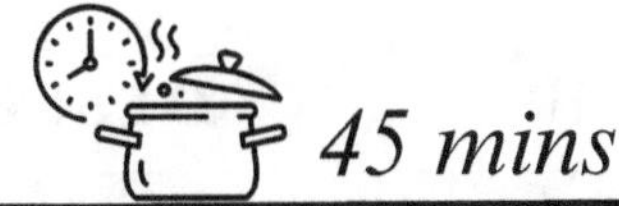 45 mins
Cook time

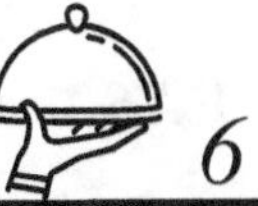 6
Servings

Ingredients

- 2 cups thinly sliced onions
- 1 cup thinly sliced and washed leek, white and light green part only
- 4 cloves garlic, thinly sliced
- 3 tablespoons extra-virgin olive oil, divided
- 2 teaspoons fresh thyme leaves
- ¼ teaspoon salt
- 2 1/2-3 pounds bone-in chicken pieces (thighs, drumsticks and/or breasts), skin removed
- ¼ cup Dijon mustard
- 2 teaspoons minced shallot
- 1 ½ teaspoons chopped fresh rosemary
- 1 teaspoon reduced-sodium soy sauce
- ¾ teaspoon freshly ground pepper

Nutrition facts per serving
Calories: 248 | Total
Carbohydrate: 8g | Dietary
Fiber: 1g | Total Sugars: 3g |
Protein: 26g | Total Fat: 12g |
Sodium: 342mg

Directions

1. Heat the oven to 400 degrees Fahrenheit.
2. In a large mixing basin, toss together the onions, leeks, garlic, 2 tablespoons oil, thyme, and salt. Spread the mixture in a 9-by-13-inch nonstick baking dish. Place the chicken breasts on the vegetables. Bake for 10 minutes at 350°F.
3. In a small mixing bowl, combine mustard, shallot, rosemary, soy sauce, and pepper; gradually whisk in the remaining 1 tablespoon oil.
4. Brush the mustard glaze over the chicken after 10 minutes. Continue baking for another 30 to 45 minutes, or until an instant-read thermometer inserted into the thickest part of a leg or breast (without contacting bone) reads 165 degrees F. Serve with the veggies.

DAILY FOOD JOURNAL

DATE:

BREAKFAST	LUNCH	DESSERT	DINNER

TODAY'S WORKOUT

WATER INTAKE

NOTES

DAILY FOOD JOURNAL

DATE:

BREAKFAST	LUNCH	DESSERT	DINNER

TODAY'S WORKOUT

WATER INTAKE

NOTES

DAILY FOOD JOURNAL

DATE:

BREAKFAST	LUNCH	DESSERT	DINNER

TODAY'S WORKOUT

WATER INTAKE

NOTES

DAILY FOOD JOURNAL

DATE:

BREAKFAST	LUNCH	DESSERT	DINNER

TODAY'S WORKOUT

WATER INTAKE

NOTES

DAILY FOOD JOURNAL

DATE:

BREAKFAST	LUNCH	DESSERT	DINNER

TODAY'S WORKOUT

WATER INTAKE

NOTES

DAILY FOOD JOURNAL

DATE:

BREAKFAST	LUNCH	DESSERT	DINNER

TODAY'S WORKOUT

WATER INTAKE

NOTES

DAILY FOOD JOURNAL

DATE:

BREAKFAST	LUNCH	DESSERT	DINNER

TODAY'S WORKOUT

WATER INTAKE

NOTES

WEEKLY PLANNER

WEEK :

MONDAY

- [ ] _______________________
- [ ] _______________________
- [ ] _______________________
- [ ] _______________________

TUESDAY

- [ ] _______________________
- [ ] _______________________
- [ ] _______________________
- [ ] _______________________

WEDNESDAY

- [ ] _______________________
- [ ] _______________________
- [ ] _______________________
- [ ] _______________________

THURSDAY

- [ ] _______________________
- [ ] _______________________
- [ ] _______________________
- [ ] _______________________

FRIDAY

- [ ] _______________________
- [ ] _______________________
- [ ] _______________________
- [ ] _______________________

SATURDAY

- [ ] _______________________
- [ ] _______________________
- [ ] _______________________
- [ ] _______________________

SUNDAY

- [ ] _______________________
- [ ] _______________________
- [ ] _______________________
- [ ] _______________________

NOTE :

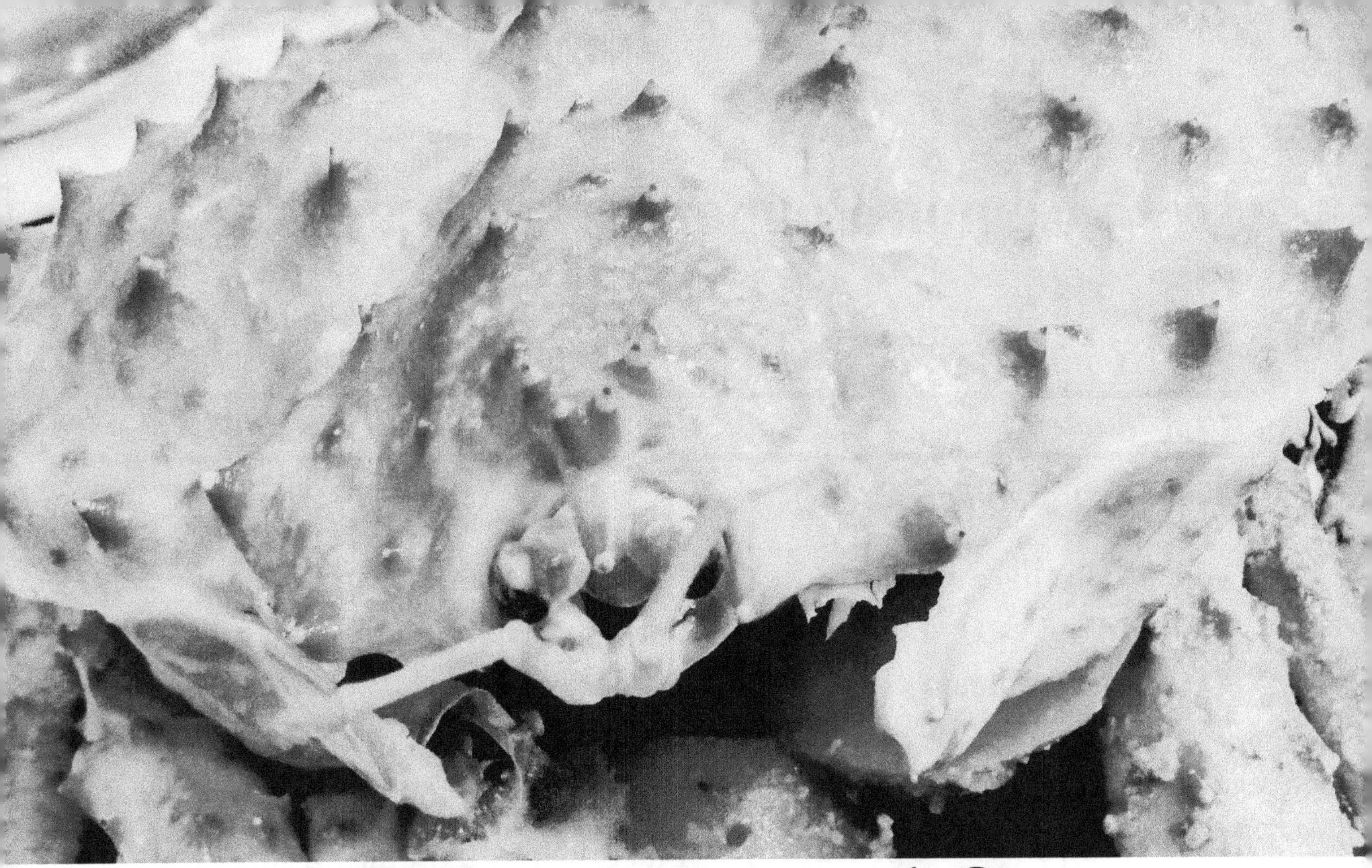

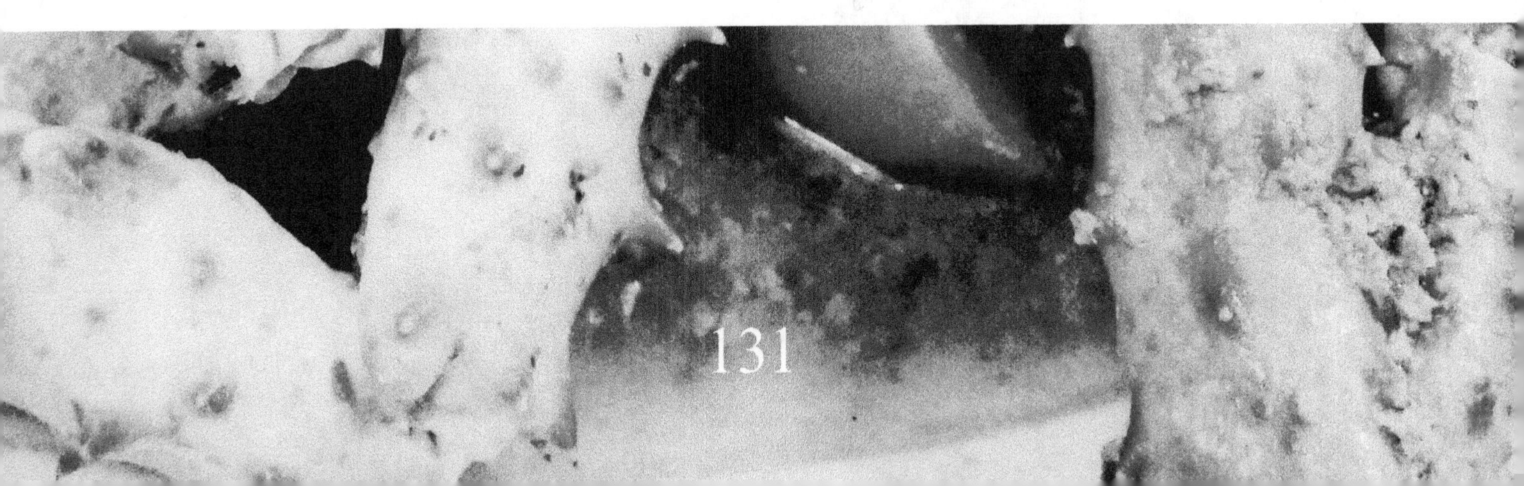

Chapter 10
Fantastic Fish and Seafood

Lemon Pepper Baked Catfish

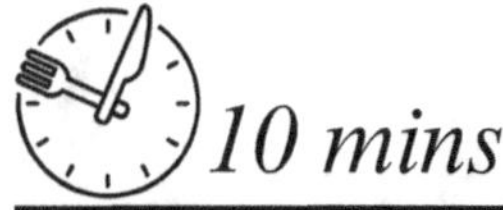 10 mins

Prep time

 20 mins

Cook time

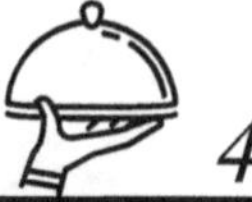 4

Servings

Ingredients

- 4 catfish fillets (about 1 pound)
- ½ cup cornmeal
- 1 tablespoon Lemon Pepper seasoning
- ½ teaspoon garlic powder
- ½ teaspoon salt

Directions

1. Mix cornmeal, lemon pepper spice, garlic powder, and salt in a shallow plate.
2. Fill the cornmeal dish with a catfish fillet. Coat thoroughly. Place them on a baking sheet that has been lined with parchment paper. Reply with the rest of the fish.
3. Cook for 20–25 minutes at 400°F, or until the fish is cooked through, golden, and flaky.

Nutrition facts per serving
Calories: 189 | Carbohydrates: 16g | Protein: 21g | Fat: 4g | Sodium: 341mg | Fiber: 2g | Sugar: 0.3g

Fish fillet in Tomato Sauce

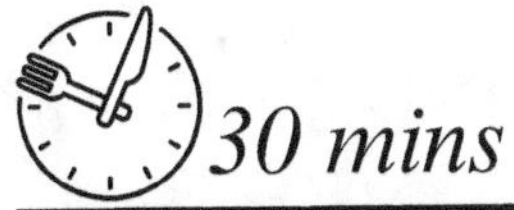 *30 mins*

Prep time

Cook time

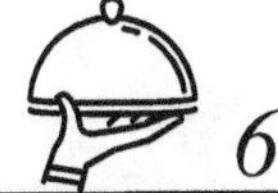 6

Servings

Ingredients

- 2 tsp ground coriander
- 2 tsp sumac
- 1 ½ tsp ground cumin
- 1 tsp dry dill weed
- 1 tsp turmeric
- 1 large yellow onion (or sweet onion), chopped
- Extra virgin olive oil
- 8 garlic cloves, chopped
- 2 jalapeno peppers, chopped (or 1 green bell pepper if you prefer mild)
- 5 medium ripe tomatoes, diced or chopped
- 3 tbsp tomato paste
- 1 lime, juice
- ½ cup water
- salt and pepper
- 2 lb cod fillet cut into large 4 to 6-ounce pieces
- ½ cup chopped fresh parsley for garnish
- 1 tbsp chopped fresh mint leaves for garnish

Directions

1. To prepare the spice mix, combine the coriander, sumac, cumin, dill, and turmeric in a small bowl. Set aside until required.

2. Heat two tablespoons of olive oil in a big skillet (with cover). Sauté the onions for 2 minutes before adding the garlic and jalapeño. Cook for another two minutes or more, stirring often, on medium-high heat, or until aromatic and golden in color.

3. Add the tomatoes and about ½ of the spice mixture now; save the remaining spice mixture for another time. Add the water, lime juice, tomato paste, salt, and pepper. Mix well to blend. After bringing to a vigorous simmer, reduce the heat to medium-low. Cook the tomato mixture, covered, for a further ten minutes, stirring now and again.

133

4. In the meantime, cover both sides of the fish fillets with the remaining ½ of the spice mixture and gently season with salt and pepper.

5. Nestle the fish pieces well in the tomato mixture after gently adding the fish fillets. Simmer for a little while on medium-high, then turn it down to medium. Once the fish is well cooked, cover and simmer for a further ten to fifteen minutes (it should be flaky).

6. Take off the heat and sprinkle the mint leaves and fresh parsley on top. Serve right now in bowls with your preferred crusty bread or Lebanese rice.

Nutrition facts per serving
Calories: 175 | Total Fat: 3g |
Sodium: 186.9mg | Total
Carbohydrate: 10.5g | Sugars:
4.7g | Protein: 28.7g

Garlic Tiger Shrimp

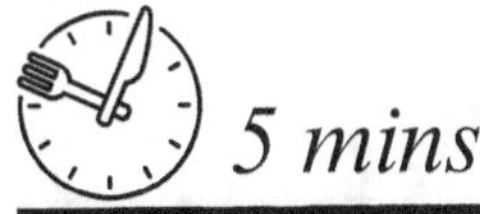 5 mins
Prep time

 6 mins
Cook time

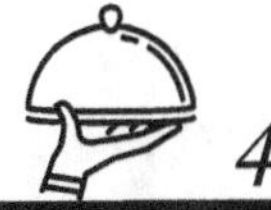 4
Servings

Ingredients

- 1 tablespoon olive oil
- 2 cloves garlic, peeled and thinly sliced
- 1/2 pound large raw shrimp (such as tiger shrimp), peeled
- Freshly chopped parsley and 1 lemon, cut into 4 wedges, to garnish

Directions

1. Preheat the oven to 400 degrees Fahrenheit. In a large, shallow ovenproof dish, combine the garlic and olive oil; cook for two to three minutes. To prevent the garlic from browning, you must keep a close eye on it.
2. Add the shrimp and toss them about in the heated oil until all of them are covered. After three more minutes, return them to the oven and continue baking until they are cooked through and pink.
3. Serve right away with some freshly cut parsley on top. Serve alongside lemon wedges for squeezing.

Nutrition facts per serving
Calories: 92 | Fat: 4g | Sodium: 80mg | Protein: 12g | Carbohydrates: 1g

Fish Tacos with Avocado Salsa

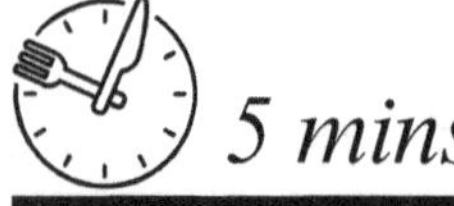 *5 mins*
Prep time

 *3 mins*
Cook time

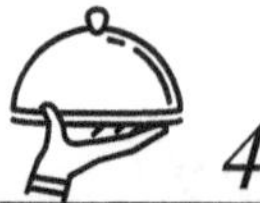 *4*
Servings

Ingredients

- 1/4 cup all-purpose flour, spooned into measuring cup and leveled (60 mL)
- 1/4 cup cornmeal (60 mL)
- 1/2 tsp onion powder (2 mL)
- 1/2 tsp chili powder
- 4 fish fillets (1 lb/500 g), such as tilapia or cod, rinsed, patted dry, and cut into 8 strips total
- 2 Tbsp canola oil
- 1/4 tsp salt
- 8 corn tortillas, warmed
- 1/2 medium avocado, peeled, pitted, and diced
- 1/2 cup fresh pico de gallo, salsa verde, or picante sauce (125 mL)
- 1 medium lime, cut into 8 wedges

Nutrition facts per serving
Calories: 375 | Fat: 14g | Fiber: 5g | Sodium: 335mg | Protein: 27g | Carbohydrates: 37g

Directions

1. In a shallow dish, mix together flour, cornmeal, onion powder, and chili powder. Apply the mixture to the fish.

2. In a big nonstick pan over medium-high heat, heat the canola oil. Fish should be added and cooked for 3 minutes on each side, or until it flakes easily with a fork. Transfer to a dish, then evenly sprinkle with salt.

3. Transfer the fish to the warmed tortillas and garnish with the same quantity of pico de gallo and avocado. Over each tortilla, squeeze a slice of lime.

Grilled Salmon with Avocado Salsa

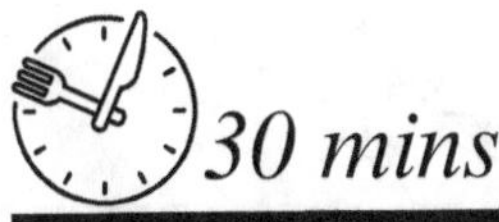 *30 mins*

Prep time

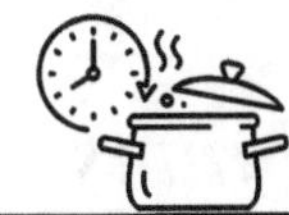

Cook time

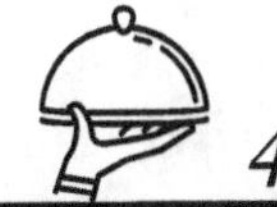 *4*

Servings

Ingredients

- 1 tablespoon olive oil
- 1 teaspoon salt
- 1 teaspoon pepper
- 1 teaspoon paprika
- 4 salmon fillets
- 2 avocados
- ¼ red onion
- 1 lime, juiced
- 1 tablespoon olive oil
- 1 ½ teaspoons salt
- cilantro, chopped for garnish(optional)

Directions

1. Combine oil, salt, pepper, and paprika in a large mixing basin. Refrigerate for 30 minutes after coating the salmon fillets with the marinade.
2. Grill the salmon for two minutes on each side on a hot 11-inch griddle pan.
3. Toss avocados, ¼ red onions, 1 tablespoon olive oil, and salt to taste in a separate bowl.
4. Top the grilled salmon with the avocado salsa. Garnish with thinly sliced cilantro.
5. Serve.

Nutrition facts per serving
Calories: 373 | Fat: 26g | Carbs: 5g | Fiber: 2g | Sugar: 0g | Protein: 25g

Grilled Shrimp Skewers

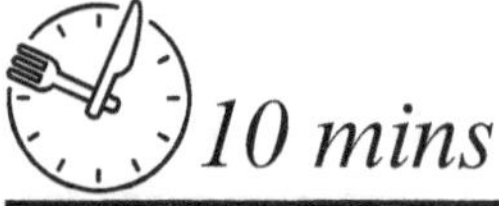 10 mins
Prep time

 5 mins
Cook time

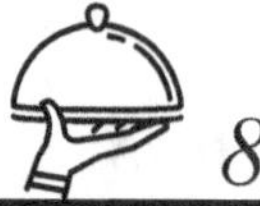 8
Servings

Ingredients

- 24 Shrimps
- 1 Red Pepper
- 1 Zucchini
- 16 Button Mushrooms
- Marinade - Optional
- Olive Oil
- Lemon
- Lemon Zest

Nutrition facts per serving
Calories: 70 | Total Fat: 1g |
Carbohydrates: 2g | Fiber: 1g |
Protein: 23g

Directions

1. Get your shrimp, red pepper, zucchini, and button mushrooms.
2. You may marinate the shrimp before grilling them to add flavor. Make a unique sauce by combining olive oil, lemon juice, and the peel of the lemon (we call it lemon zest). Add the shrimp to the sauce. Allow them to soak up the delectable flavors.
3. Place your marinated large shrimp on the wooden skewers. You may also use metal skewers. Between the shrimp, layer red pepper, zucchini, and mushrooms. For each skewer, use two to three big shrimp.
4. Warm up a grill or grill pan. It will reduce the time spent on the grill. Place your shrimp skewers on the grill. Cook the skewers for at least 2 to 3 minutes on each side, depending on the size of the shrimp.
5. When the shrimp are done and properly cooked, they will turn pink and no longer be see-through. Shrimp cooks rapidly, so don't overcook them.

Baked salmon with mayonnaise

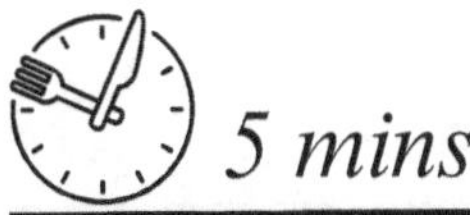 **5 mins**
Prep time

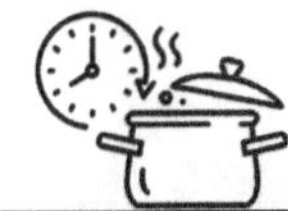 **10 mins**
Cook time

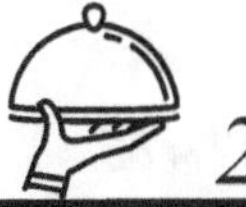 *2*
Servings

Ingredients

- 12 oz (12 oz) salmon fillets 2 x 180g , skin off
- 3 broccoli florets
- (1/4) zucchini, sliced
- salt and pepper
- 2 tablespoons mayonnaise
- 1 teaspoon garlic finely minced
- 4 slices lemon
- 2 tsp capers
- 1/2 green onion sliced thinly
- 6-8 thin chili slices

Nutrition facts per serving
Calories: 363 | Carbohydrates: 3g | Protein: 37g | Fat: 22g | Sodium: 227mg | Fiber: 1g | Sugar: 1g

Directions

1. Turn the oven on to 180°C/400°F.
2. Fold two large sheets of foil in half so that they envelop the salmon fillets. top with salmon and arrange broccoli and zucchini in the center of the foil. Add a dash of pepper and salt.
3. In a small bowl, mix together the mayonnaise and garlic. put aside
4. Add lemon, capers, chili, green onions, and garlic mayonnaise to the salmon's top. Seal the salmon by folding the foil.
5. Preheat the oven to 8 to 10 degrees. Take it out of the oven and make sure it's done enough. accompany a crisp salad and more mayonnaise or aioli. Add plenty of black pepper and salt flakes for seasoning.

Tuna Salad lettuce wraps

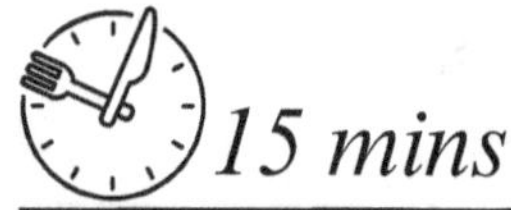 *15 mins*

 *2*

Prep time   *Cook time*   *Servings*

Ingredients

- 2 cans (5 ounces each) of tuna, drained
- ¼ cup mayonnaise
- 2 ribs celery, finely diced
- 1 English cucumber, finely diced
- 1 shallot, finely diced
- 2 tablespoons chopped parsley
- 1 tablespoon Dijon mustard
- 1 tablespoon lemon juice
- ½ teaspoon sea salt
- ½ teaspoon paprika
- ¼ teaspoon garlic powder
- ¼ teaspoon ground black pepper
- 8 to 10 leaves of Romaine lettuce or butter lettuce
- Optional toppings - sesame seeds, sliced green onions, chopped parsley or other soft herbs like dill or cilantro

Nutrition facts per serving
Calories: 360 | Total fat: 22g |
Sodium: 980mg | Carbs: 14g |
Fiber: 4g | Sugar: 6g | Protein:
28g

Directions

1. In a large bowl, combine the tuna, mayonnaise, mustard, sugar, paprika, garlic powder, black pepper, chopped bell pepper, chopped celery, chopped shallot, chopped parsley, and lemon juice. Stir until well blended.
2. Put a spoonful into each lettuce leaf.
3. Serve right away after adding your preferred toppings.

Grilled Tuna Steaks with Cilantro and Basil

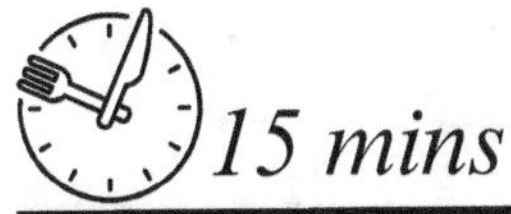 15 mins

Prep time

 3 mins

Cook time

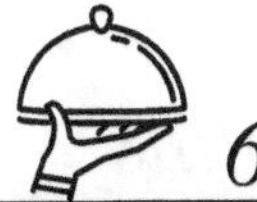 6

Servings

Ingredients

- 3 tablespoons light soy sauce
- 3 tablespoons canola oil
- 1/4 teaspoon red pepper flakes
- 6 tuna steaks (rinsed, patted dry)
- canola oil cooking spray
- 1/2 cup chopped, fresh cilantro leaves
- 1/4 cup chopped, fresh basil leaves
- 2 tablespoons fresh lime juice
- 1 tablespoon white vinegar
- 1/2 teaspoon minced garlic

Nutrition facts per serving
Calories: 210 | Total Fat: 10.0g |
Sodium: 240mg | Total
Carbohydrate: 2g | Dietary
Fiber: 0g | Sugars: 1g | Protein:
27g

Directions

1. Combine the soy sauce, pepper flakes, and canola oil in a small bowl. Put the tuna steaks in a big plastic bag that can be sealed, along with 2 tablespoons of the soy sauce mixture. To coat the tuna steaks, turn the bag several times. Keep chilled for no more than half an hour.

2. Heat up the cooking spray-coated grill to a high temperature. Meanwhile, mix the cilantro, basil, lime juice, vinegar, and garlic in a separate small bowl.

3. After taking the tuna out of the bag and throwing away any remaining marinade, grill it for 1 1/2 minutes on each side, or until the interior temperature reaches 145 °F. Tuna will turn rough if it is overcooked.

4. Top with equal parts of the cilantro mixture, and serve with the remaining soy sauce mixture.

141

One-Pot Garlic Shrimp & Broccoli

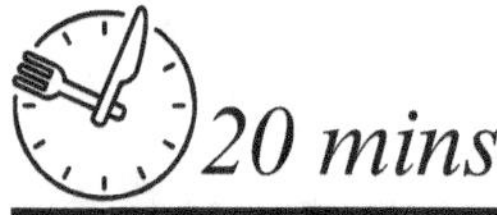 *20 mins*

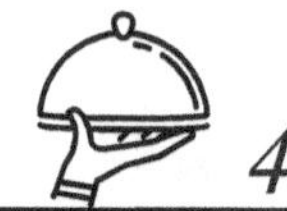 *4*

Prep time   *Cook time*   *Servings*

Ingredients

- 3 tablespoons extra-virgin olive oil, divided
- 6 medium cloves garlic, sliced, divided
- 4 cups small broccoli florets
- ½ cup diced red bell pepper
- ½ teaspoon salt, divided
- ½ teaspoon ground pepper, divided
- 1 pound peeled and deveined raw shrimp
- 2 teaspoons lemon juice, plus more to taste

Nutrition facts per serving
Calories: 214 | Total
Carbohydrate: 6g | Dietary
Fiber: 2g | Total Sugars: 2g |
Protein: 25g | Total Fat: 11g |
Sodium: 441mg

Directions

1. Heat 2 tablespoons of oil in a large saucepan over medium heat. Cook until half of the garlic starts to brown, about 1 minute. Add the broccoli, bell pepper, and 1/4 teaspoon salt and pepper.
2. Cook, stirring once or twice and adding 1 tablespoon water if the saucepan is too dry, until the veggies are soft, 3 to 5 minutes. Keep heated in a dish.
3. Increase the heat to medium-high and add the remaining 1 tablespoon of oil to the saucepan. Cook until the remaining garlic starts to brown, approximately 1 minute.
4. Cook, tossing constantly, until the shrimp are barely cooked through, 3 to 5 minutes. Return the broccoli mixture to the saucepan, along with the lemon juice, and stir to blend.

Poached cod with tomato basil sauce

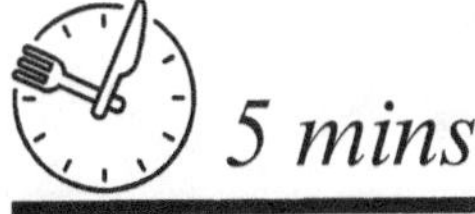 5 mins
Prep time

 25 mins
Cook time

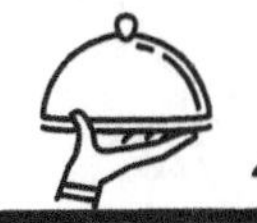 4
Servings

Ingredients

- 4 - 6 oz frozen white fish fillets of your choice
- 2 cups cherry tomatoes, cut in half
- 2 cloves garlic, finely sliced
- 1/2 cup light chicken stock
- 1/4 cup dry white wine (or use more chicken stock)
- 1/2 tsp salt, I use Himalayan salt
- 1/2 tsp ground black pepper
- 1/4 cup fresh basil leaves, finely chopped (plus more for garnish)

Directions

1. In a saucé pan over medium heat, combine the tomatoes, garlic, salt, and pepper. Cook for 5 minutes, or until the tomatoes begin to soften and blister.

2. Add the chopped basil, frozen fish fillets, white wine (if using), and chicken stock. After the fish is cooked through, simmer it for 20 to 25 minutes.

3. Serve over quinoa, couscous, or rice, if preferred, and garnish with a few more handfuls of finely chopped basil.

Nutrition facts per serving
Calories: 185 | Carbohydrates: 6g | Protein: 32g | Fat: 2g | Sodium: 438mg | Fiber: 1g | Sugar: 3g

Steamed Asian white fish

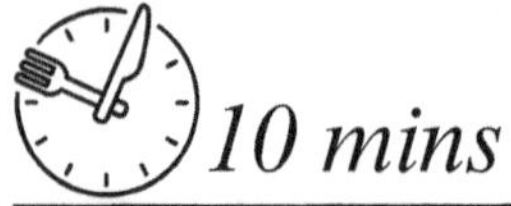 *10 mins*

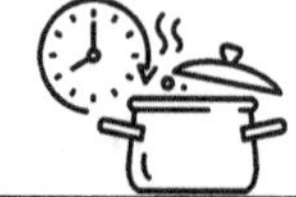 *10 mins*

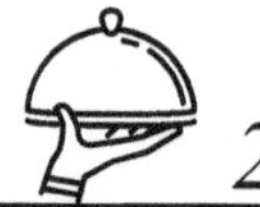 2

| Prep time | Cook time | Servings |

Ingredients

- 3 slices daikon radish peeled and sliced thin
- 10 ounces white fish boneless and skinless fillets (cod, tilapia, halibut)
- 1 inch ginger fresh ginger knob peeled and cut into thin slabs
- 2 bok choy optional - cut in half lengthwise or veggie of choice

Asian sauce

- ¾ teaspoon dashi powder mixed in ¼ cup water (or ¼ cup homemade dashi broth)
- ¼ cup water to mix with dried dashi powder (hold if using homemade dashi broth)
- 1 tablespoon oil

Directions

1. Place enough water in the bottom of the pan to keep the water level at least 2 inches away from the steamer plate, etc. Turn on your heat and bring your steamer to a boil.

2. Place peeled and sliced daikon slices (or other veggies such as carrot slices or lettuce) on your steaming plate to keep the fish from sticking to the plate or steamer basket.

3. Place cod fillets (or other mild white fish of choice), on top of the daikon radishes (or other veggies) on your steaming platter (bamboo basket).

4. Place julienne-cut ginger on top of fish fillets (if using the entire fish, pack the cavity with ginger slices). Just a quick reminder that you will need additional ginger julienne pieces for the Asian sauce.

- 3 cloves garlic peeled and minced
- 6 green onions cut into thirds and sliced horizontally
- 2 tablespoon mirin (Japanese cooking rice wine)
- 1 teaspoon sugar or sugar alternative
- 2 tablespoon soy sauce or tamari to keep gluten free
- ⅛ teaspoon white pepper or to taste
- sesame oil - 1 teaspoon
- 1 bunch cilantro (coriander) optional but very delicious
- Cauliflower Rice, mushrooms, veggies - optional

Nutrition facts per serving
Calories: 338 | Carbohydrates: 22g | Protein: 42g | Fat: 11g | Fiber: 9g | Sugar: 10g

5. Arrange bok choy or other green veggies of choice around the fish. Place the fish with the bok choy dish in the steamer once the water in the steamer comes to a boil. Depending on the size of your fish, you will need to stream it for 4 to 10 minutes. Larger or thicker fish fillets or entire fish will take longer to cook than thinner fillets. Our cod was done in 4 minutes. Your fish should flake easily with a fork and no longer be transparent. The rapidly cooked green vegetables should be al dente.

6. In the meantime, prepare your Asian sauce. In a small saucepan, combine the oil, ginger, garlic, half of the green onions, dashi broth, mirin, sugar or sugar substitute, soy or tamari sauce, and white pepper to taste. Season to taste. Just before removing the sauce from the pan, toss in the remaining green onions.

7. Drain the fish and bok choy from the steamer. Drizzle Asian sauce and sesame oil over top. Garnish with cilantro (coriander) and serve! Serve it alone for a low-carb supper or with rice for a filling, complete meal.

Chapter 11
Main Dish, sauce and dressing

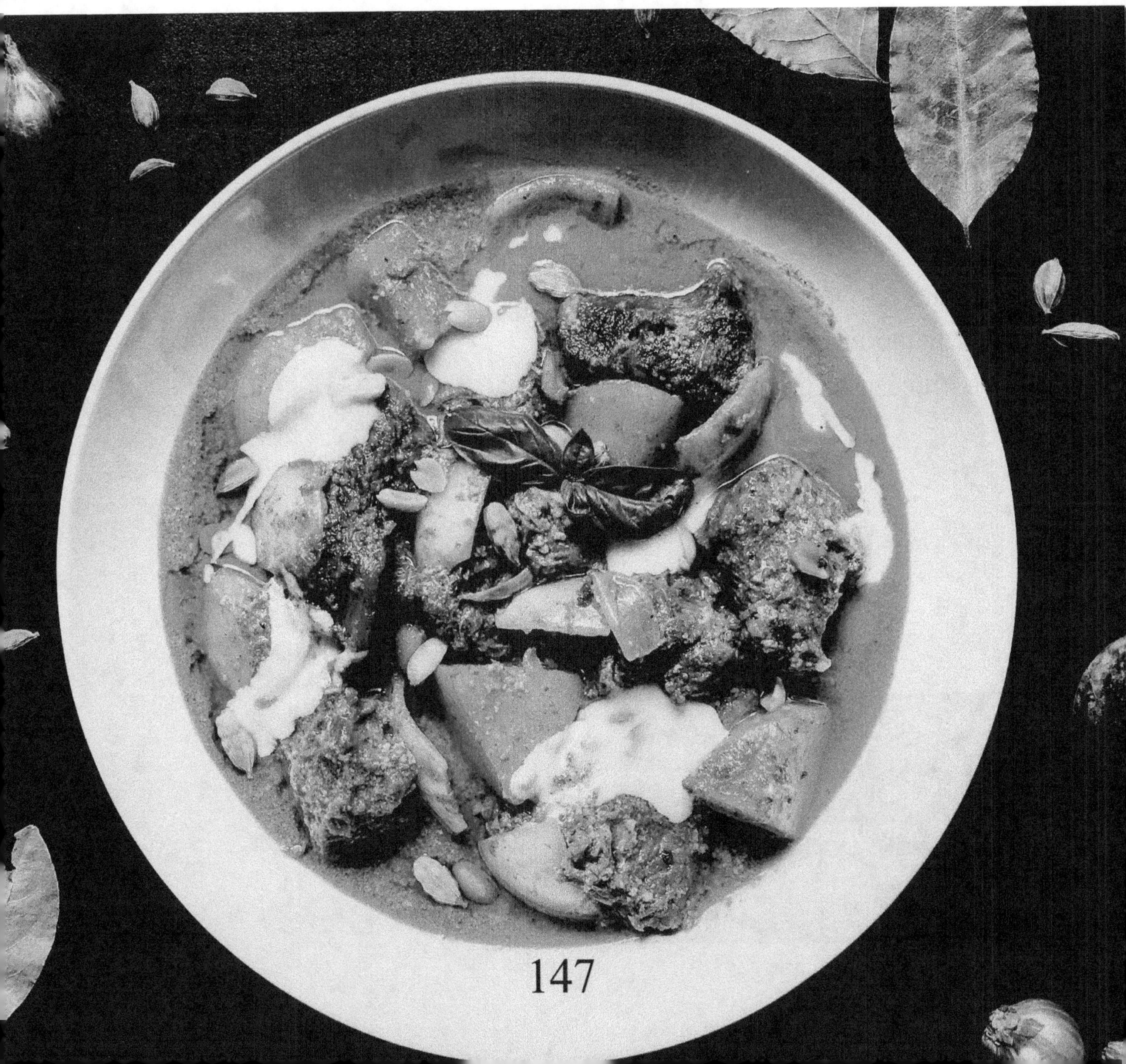

147

Avocado Cilantro Sauce

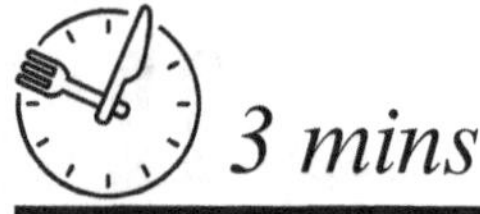 *3 mins*

Prep time

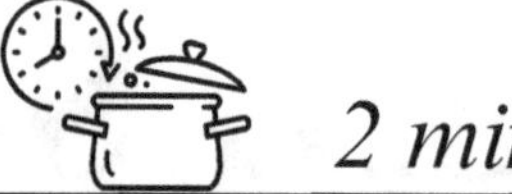 *2 mins*

Cook time

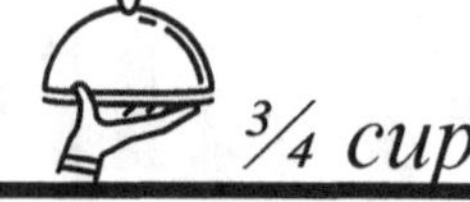 *¾ cup*

Servings

Ingredients

- Half an avocado
- 1/4 cup Greek yogurt
- 1/2 cup water (more as needed to adjust consistency)
- 1 cup cilantro leaves and stems
- 1 small clove of garlic
- 1/2 teaspoon salt
- A squeeze of lime juice

Directions

1. In a food processor or blender, combine all of the ingredients and blend until smooth.

Nutrition facts per serving
Calories: 70 | Total Fat: 5g |
Sodium: 300mg | Total
Carbohydrates: 6g | Dietary
Fiber: 2g | Sugars: 1g | Protein:
2g

Asian Hot Mustard

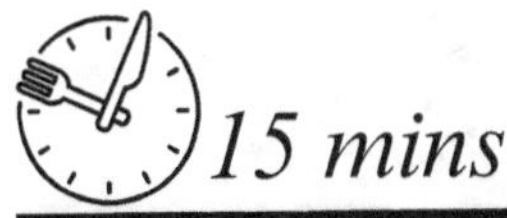 *15 mins*
Prep time

Cook time

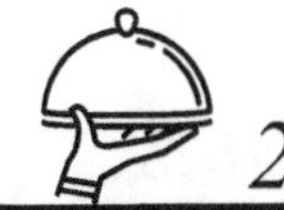 *2*
Servings

Ingredients

- 1 tablespoon mustard powder
- ⅛ teaspoon salt
- ⅛ teaspoon white pepper
- 1½ teaspoon hot water
- ½ teaspoon vegetable oil
- ½ teaspoon rice vinegar
- 1/4 teaspoon granulated sugar (optional)

Nutrition facts per serving
Calories: 13 | Carbohydrates: 1g | Protein: 1g | Fat: 1g | Sodium: 73mg | Fiber: 1g | Sugar: 1g

Directions

1. In a small mixing basin, add the dry ingredients and stir until well incorporated. Stir in the water until a liquid paste develops and all dry ingredients are absorbed. Stir in the oil and vinegar until thoroughly mixed.

2. Allow your spicy mustard to rest for 10 minutes, covered, before re-stirring to ensure the dry components are completely absorbed. At this stage, taste and modify it to your liking.

3. If you like a thinner consistency, add additional water or oil. If you like it a little tarter, add extra vinegar. If you want it hotter, omit the vinegar entirely, as vinegar dulls the flavor of the mustard. If you want it spicy, add extra white pepper and/or mustard powder. If you wish to lessen the harshness of the dried mustard, add honey.

Veggie Stir-fry with Tofu

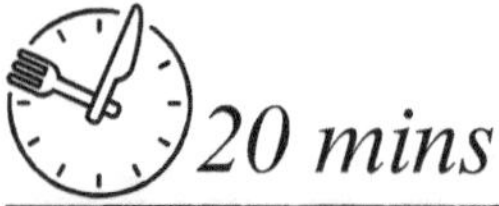 20 mins

 30 mins

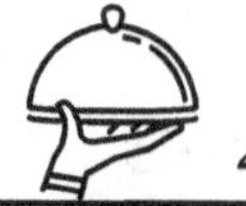 4

| Prep time | Cook time | Servings |

Ingredients

For Tofu
- 1 (14-oz.) block extra-firm tofu, fresh or frozen and defrosted
- 1 tbsp. low-sodium soy sauce
- 1 tbsp. sesame oil
- 1/2 tsp. freshly ground black pepper
- 2 tbsp. cornstarch

For the Stir-fry
- 3 tbsp. extra-virgin olive oil, divided
- Kosher salt
- 3 cloves garlic, minced
- 1 tbsp. freshly minced ginger
- 8 oz. string beans, trimmed
- 2 small carrots, sliced
- 1 small head broccoli, cut into florets
- 1 red bell pepper, seeded and sliced
- 2 green onions, thinly sliced

Directions

1. Tofu should be cooked for 2 minutes in a medium saucepan of salted, boiling water. Simmer until the tofu has thoroughly defrosted, if using frozen tofu. Allow to drain in a colander lined with paper towels after removing from the heat.

2. Gently squeeze and pat dry when it is cool enough to handle. If using frozen tofu, squeeze off the water with more force.

3. Toss tofu with soy sauce, sesame oil, and black pepper in a medium mixing basin. Toss tofu with cornstarch once the liquids have been absorbed.

4. Heat 2 tablespoons of oil in a large pan over medium-high heat. Cook until brown on all sides, 7 to 8 minutes. Season with salt and pepper and set aside.

For the sauce

- 2 tbsp. low-sodium soy sauce
- 2 tsp. sesame oil
- 1/4 c. water
- 2 tbsp. packed brown sugar
- 2 tsp. cornstarch

5. Cook until aromatic, 1 minute, with the remaining 1 tablespoon of oil. String beans, carrots, broccoli, red pepper, and green onions should be added at the end. Cook until the vegetables are soft, 8 to 10 minutes. Season with salt and pepper, if desired.

6. Combine the soy sauce, sesame oil, water, brown sugar, and cornstarch in a small mixing dish. Return to the skillet with the tofu and sauce mixture. Stir and heat for 2 minutes, or until slightly thickened.

Nutrition facts per serving
Calories: 345 | Fat: 21g |
Sodium: 905mg |
Carbohydrates: 24g | Fiber: 7g |
Sugar: 14g | Protein: 14g

Apple Cider Vinaigrette

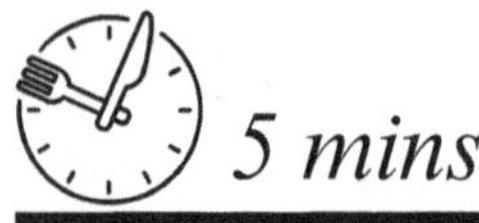 *5 mins*

Prep time

Cook time

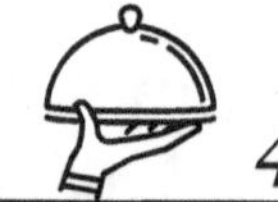 *4*

Servings

Ingredients

- 1/3 cup olive oil
- 1/4 cup apple cider vinegar
- 1 tablespoon honey
- 1 teaspoon Dijon mustard
- 1 clove garlic, minced
- Salt and pepper , to taste

Directions

1. Whisk together all of the ingredients in a small bowl.
2. Pour into a serving jar and serve, or refrigerate in an airtight container.

Nutrition facts per serving
Calories: 180 | Carbs: 5g |
Protein: 1g | Fat: 18g | Sodium:
16mg | Fiber: 1g | Sugar: 4g

Roasted Red Pepper Sauce

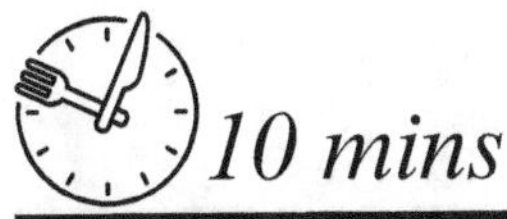 *10 mins*
Prep time

 *1 hr*
Cook time

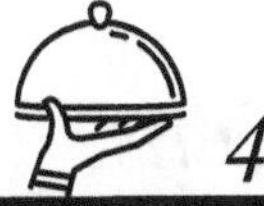 *4*
Servings

Ingredients

- 2 red peppers
- 1 ½ tbsp olive oil
- 1 small garlic clove, crushed
- 1 small shallot, roughly chopped
- 85 ml vegetable stock
- ½ tsp sugar, to taste (optional)

Nutrition facts per serving
Calories: 62 | Fat: 4g | Carbs: 5g | Sugar: 5g | Fiber: 1g | Protein: 1g | Sodium: 0.03g

Directions

1. Preheat the oven to 200°C/180°C. Place the peppers on a baking sheet and roast for 45 minutes, or until the skins are browned. Remove from the oven and place in a plastic bag to sweat, allowing the skins to fall off more easily.

2. When the skins are cold enough to handle, pull them off with your fingers. Open the peppers, remove and discard the seeds and membrane, and then coarsely cut the red meat.

3. In a skillet, heat the olive oil. Fry the garlic and shallots for a few minutes until the oil is heated. Continue to cook for a few minutes, stirring constantly, until everything is combined. Bring the vegetable stock to a boil, then let it reduce slightly.

4. Blend the contents of the pan until smooth in a blender. Season with salt and pepper to taste. Depending on how ripe the peppers are, you shouldn't need any sugar, but if they still have a somewhat bitter flavor, return the sauce to the pan, add sugar to taste, and let it dissolve over heat. Serve immediately or at room temperature.

Pineapple Chicken Stir Fry

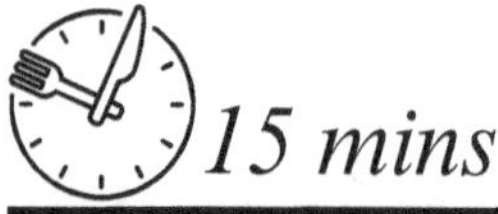 *15 mins*
Prep time

 *25 mins*
Cook time

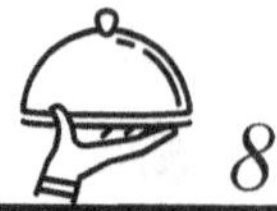 *8*
Servings

Ingredients

- 2 tbsp avocado oil
- 1.5 lb raw chicken breasts, diced
- 1 small red onion, diced
- 1 red pepper, diced
- 1 yellow pepper, diced
- 1 small head broccoli, chopped into small florets
- 20 oz can pineapple chunks
- Sesame seeds
- 1/4 cup pineapple juice (from can with chunks)
- 1/4 cup rice wine vinegar
- 1/3 cup soy sauce (tamari if GF)
- 1.5 tsp sesame oil
- 2 tbsp arrowroot powder (or cornstarch)

Nutrition facts per serving
Calories: 274 | Total Fat: 7.1g | Sodium: 345.6mg | Total Carbohydrate: 31.4g | Sugars: 21.9g | Protein: 22.9g

Directions

1. Heat 1 tablespoon of avocado oil in a large skillet. Cook for 7-8 minutes, or until the chicken is cooked through.
2. Remove from the pan and set aside to drain any extra liquid.
3. Add another tablespoon of avocado oil to the same skillet, along with the onion, peppers, and broccoli. Cook for another 7-8 minutes, or until the vegetables begin to soften.
4. Meanwhile, mix together all of the sauce ingredients.
5. When the vegetables are done, return the chicken to the pan with the sauce and pineapple pieces.
6. Cook for 5–6 minutes over medium heat, or until the sauce has thickened.
7. Sprinkle with sesame seeds, and serve over rice! Enjoy.

Sheet-Pan Chicken Fajita Bowls

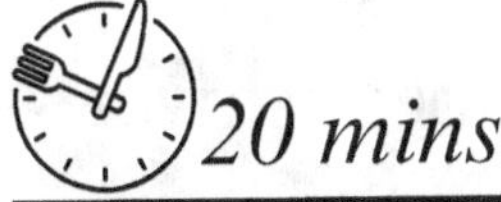 20 mins
Prep time

 20 mins
Cook time

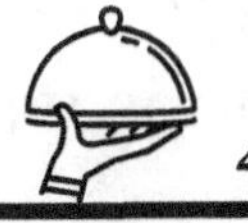 4
Servings

Ingredients

- 2 teaspoons chili powder
- 2 teaspoons ground cumin
- ¾ teaspoon salt, divided
- ½ teaspoon garlic powder
- ½ teaspoon smoked paprika
- ¼ teaspoon ground pepper
- 2 tablespoons olive oil, divided
- 1 ¼ pounds chicken tenders
- 1 medium yellow onion, sliced
- 1 medium red bell pepper, sliced
- 1 medium green bell pepper, sliced
- 4 cups chopped stemmed kale
- 1 (15 ounce) can no-salt-added black beans, rinse

Directions

1. Preheat the oven to 425°F with a big rimmed baking sheet.
2. In a large mixing bowl, whisk together the chili powder, cumin, 1/2 teaspoon salt, garlic powder, paprika, and ground pepper. Set aside 1 teaspoon of the spice mixture in a medium mixing dish. In the big mixing bowl, combine 1 tablespoon of oil with the remaining spice combination. Toss in the chicken, onion, red and green bell peppers, and parsley.
3. Remove the baking sheet from the oven and spray it with cooking spray. Spread the chicken mixture on the pan in an equal layer. Bake for 15 minutes at 350°F.
4. Meanwhile, in a large mixing bowl, toss the kale and black beans with the remaining 1/4 teaspoon salt and 1 tablespoon olive oil to coat.

155

- ¼ cup low-fat plain Greek yogurt
- 1 tablespoon lime juice
- 2 teaspoons water

5. Take the baking sheet out of the oven. Combine the chicken and veggies in a large mixing bowl. Evenly distribute the greens and beans over top. 5 to 7 minutes of roasting time, or until the chicken is cooked through and the veggies are tender.

6. Meanwhile, whisk together the reserved spice mixture, yogurt, lime juice, and water.

7. Divide the chicken-vegetable combination into four serving dishes. Serve with the yogurt dressing.

Nutrition facts per serving
Calories: 343 | Total Carbohydrate 24g | Dietary Fiber: 8g | Total Sugars: 4g | Protein: 43g | Total Fat: 10g | Sodium: 605mg

Low Carb Zucchini Lasagna

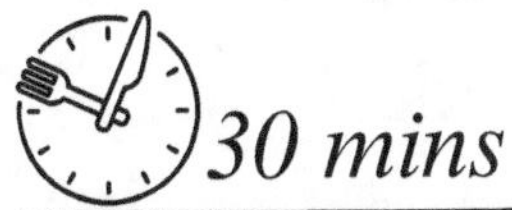 30 mins

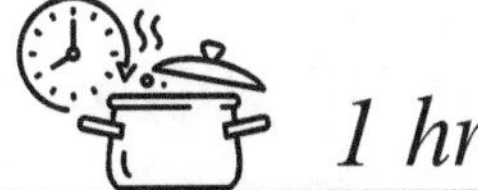 1 hr

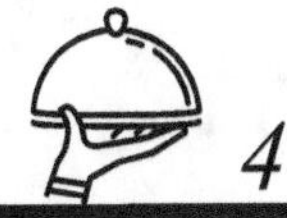 4

Prep time — *Cook time* — *Servings*

Ingredients

- 16 oz. ground beef, (92% lean)
- 2 medium zucchini
- 4½ oz. onion
- 2 cloves garlic
- 1 serrano chili
- 3 tomatoes
- 5½ oz. mushrooms
- ½ cube Knorr chicken bouillon
- ½ cup shredded low-fat mozzarella
- 1 teaspoon paprika
- 1 teaspoon dried thyme
- 1 teaspoon dried basil
- Salt & pepper
- Cooking spray

Nutrition facts per serving
Calories: 244 | Fat: 7.9g |
Sodium 558.4mg |
Carbohydrates: 12.3g | Fiber:
3.6g | Sugar: 6.3g | Protein:
30.4g

Directions

1. Cut the zucchini into 12-inch (1 cm) pieces with a julienne peeler. Set aside for 10 minutes after lightly seasoning with salt.
2. Using a paper towel, blot the zucchini slices. Grill or broil them for 3 minutes on high heat in the oven.
3. Place the zucchini on paper towels after grilling or broiling to absorb as much moisture as possible.
4. Remove the ends of the tomatoes. Place them in boiling water for a few minutes, then rinse with cold water and peel off the skin. You may also use canned tomatoes instead.
5. Chop the onions, garlic, chiles, peeled tomatoes, and mushrooms coarsely.
6. In a large pan, coat with cooking spray and sauté the garlic, onion, and chile for 1 minute.

7. Add the tomatoes and mushrooms to the skillet and cook for an additional 4 minutes. Then remove it from the heat and set it aside.

8. Cook the meat and paprika in the same pan as the vegetables until well browned.

9. Return the veggies to the skillet, followed by the chicken bouillon and other seasonings. Allow the sauce to boil on low heat for 25 minutes.

10. Preheat the oven to 375°F (190°C). Line a small baking pan with parchment paper and arrange 1/3 of the zucchini at the bottom. Place a third of the beef sauce on top. Continue layering zucchini until you've used up all of the sauce and zucchini.

11. Bake for 35 minutes, then top with shredded mozzarella. Remove the lasagna from the oven and set it aside for 10 minutes before serving.

DAILY FOOD JOURNAL

DATE:

BREAKFAST	LUNCH	DESSERT	DINNER

TODAY'S WORKOUT

WATER INTAKE

NOTES

DAILY FOOD JOURNAL

DATE:

BREAKFAST	LUNCH	DESSERT	DINNER

TODAY'S WORKOUT

WATER INTAKE

NOTES

DAILY FOOD JOURNAL

DATE:

BREAKFAST	LUNCH	DESSERT	DINNER

TODAY'S WORKOUT

WATER INTAKE

NOTES

DAILY FOOD JOURNAL

DATE:

BREAKFAST	LUNCH	DESSERT	DINNER

TODAY'S WORKOUT

WATER INTAKE

NOTES

DAILY FOOD JOURNAL

DATE:

BREAKFAST	LUNCH	DESSERT	DINNER

TODAY'S WORKOUT

WATER INTAKE

NOTES

DAILY FOOD JOURNAL

DATE:

BREAKFAST	LUNCH	DESSERT	DINNER

TODAY'S WORKOUT

WATER INTAKE

NOTES

DAILY FOOD JOURNAL

DATE:

BREAKFAST	LUNCH	DESSERT	DINNER

TODAY'S WORKOUT

WATER INTAKE

NOTES

WEEKLY PLANNER

WEEK :

MONDAY

- [ ] ______________________
- [ ] ______________________
- [ ] ______________________
- [ ] ______________________

TUESDAY

- [ ] ______________________
- [ ] ______________________
- [ ] ______________________
- [ ] ______________________

WEDNESDAY

- [ ] ______________________
- [ ] ______________________
- [ ] ______________________
- [ ] ______________________

THURSDAY

- [ ] ______________________
- [ ] ______________________
- [ ] ______________________
- [ ] ______________________

FRIDAY

- [ ] ______________________
- [ ] ______________________
- [ ] ______________________
- [ ] ______________________

SATURDAY

- [ ] ______________________
- [ ] ______________________
- [ ] ______________________
- [ ] ______________________

SUNDAY

- [ ] ______________________
- [ ] ______________________
- [ ] ______________________
- [ ] ______________________

NOTE :

CHAPTER 12: TIPS FOR SUCCESS

As we come to the end of our adventure through the realms of "Diabetic diet after 50," it's critical to remember that this isn't a passing fad. It's a commitment to a way of life that goes beyond the pages of this book—to your health, energy, and the pure joy of living life to the fullest.

Maintaining a healthy lifestyle is a gift to your future self, not a duty. Here are some of the reasons why this commitment is as ageless as it is valuable:

- Consistency is essential. Health is a journey, not a destination. A sustainable and thriving lifestyle is built on consistency in your nutritional choices, physical exercise, and self-care rituals.
- Adaptability is important. Life, like our bodies, is dynamic. Be open to changing your approach as you elegantly traverse the years beyond 50. It's natural for your nutritional demands, exercise levels, and general health practices to change.
- Embracing Physical Activity: A healthy lifestyle requires regular exercise. It's not about going to extremes; it's about finding hobbies that make you happy and keep you active. Make it a part of your everyday routine, whether it's a daily stroll, mild yoga, or dancing in your living room.

- Mindful Eating as a Ritual: Eating is more than simply nourishment for your body; it's also a sensory experience. Cultivate attentive eating habits—savor each meal, enjoy the tastes, and be present in the moment. This not only improves your eating satisfaction but also promotes healthy digestion.

- Water is the elixir of life; therefore, drink plenty of it. Keep hydrated to help your body's many processes. It's a simple yet effective practice that helps with general well-being.

- Check-ins with healthcare providers on a regular basis: Regular health check-ups are not only for resolving problems; they are also preventative actions. Maintain contact with your healthcare team, address any changes in your health, and verify that your diabetes management plan meets your changing requirements.

- Stress Management: Life is full of problems, but how we respond to them counts. Blood sugar levels can be affected by stress. Find hobbies that help you relax, such as reading, gardening, or spending time with family and friends.

- Quality Sleep: Adequate and restorative sleep is essential for optimal health. Create a relaxing sleeping environment, and prioritize the rest your body requires to recuperate.

- Celebrating Small-Scale Victories: Health is multifaceted. It's not only about the weight on the scale. Celebrate tiny triumphs, whether they be an increase in energy, a newfound passion for a vegetable, or the pleasure of cooking a great and diabetes-friendly meal.

- Enjoy the journey: Remember that this is your journey to enjoy. Find delight in the tiny things, enjoy the flavors of each day, and appreciate your body's and spirit's resiliency.

As we come to the end of our journey, I want you to see it as a new beginning—the start of a bright and healthy chapter in your life. The ideas presented in this book are not rules, but rather powerful recommendations. Accept them with the same zeal that you've shown for every previous milestone along your incredible adventure.

Dear Valued Readers,

his journey through the pages of "Diabetic Diet After 50" has been as enriching for you as it has been for me. Your feedback is invaluable! If you found the book insightful, please take a moment to leave a review. Your thoughts can guide others on their path to healthier living.

Additionally, if you'd like to stay connected and receive updates on future releases, please follow my Author Central page. Your support means the world to me.

For any personal messages or queries, feel free to reach out via email at michellerockwell98@yahoo.com . I look forward to hearing from you and am grateful for the opportunity to share this transformative journey with you.

Thank you for being a part of this community of wellness and wisdom.

Warm regards,
Michelle Rockwell.